# A PRIMER ON LIMB PROSTHETICS

## ABOUT THE AUTHOR

**A. Bennett Wilson Jr.** is a mechanical engineer who joined the staff of the National Academy of Sciences in 1949 to assist in the development and coordination of a nationwide research and development program in artificial limbs. He served as Executive Director of the Committee on Prosthetics Research and Development of the NAS, as the program came to be known, from 1960-1975. He is a founding member and fellow of the International Society for Prosthetics and Orthotics and also a founding member of Technical Committee 168 (Limb Prosthetics and Orthotics of the International Standards Organization). Mr. Wilson was involved in initiation of current education programs in prosthetics and orthotics and in the introduction of many new devices and techniques in the field of physical rehabilitation.

# A PRIMER ON LIMB PROSTHETICS

*By*

**A. BENNETT WILSON, JR., B.S.M.E.**

*Formerly, Associate Professor*
*Department of Orthopedic Surgery and Rehabilitation*
*Medical School, University of Virginia*

CHARLES C THOMAS • PUBLISHER, LTD.
*Springfield • Illinois • U.S.A.*

*Published and Distributed Throughout the World by*
CHARLES C THOMAS • PUBLISHER, LTD.
2600 South First Street
Springfield, Illinois 62794-9265


ISBN 0-398-06900-X (cloth)
ISBN 0-398-06897-6 (paper)

Library of Congress Catalog Card Number: 98-28843

*With* THOMAS BOOKS *careful attention is given to all details of manufacturing and design. It is the Publisher's desire to present books that are satisfactory as to their physical qualities and artistic possibilities and appropriate for their particular use.* THOMAS BOOKS *will be true to those laws of quality that assure a good name and good will.*

*Printed in the United States of America*
*CR-R-3*

*Library of Congress Cataloging-in-Publication Data*

Wilson, A. Bennett
A primer on limb prosthetics / by A. Bennett Wilson, Jr.
p. cm.
Includes bibliographical references and index.
ISBN 0-398-06900-X (cloth) ISBN 0-398-06897-6 (paper).
1. Artificial limbs. 2. Amputees--Rehabilitation. I. Title.
(DNLM: 1. Artificial Limbs. 2. Prosthesis Fitting.
3. Amputation--rehabilitation. WE 172W746p 1998)
RD 756.W585 1998
617.5'80592--dc21
DNLM/DLC 98-28843
for Library of Congress CIP

# FOREWORD

The purpose of this book is stated clearly in the Preface and amply fulfilled by the author. Through a long and honored association with the field of prosthetics and orthotics, Ben Wilson has worked to shape events and to better the lot of the patients served. This vantage point has given him the opportunity to observe events and developments. He has shared the results with the reader in a clear and lucid style.

The intended audience should find this book of tremendous assistance in understanding a field that is oftentimes portrayed in a confused and sensationalized fashion by the popular media and frequently glossed over in most professional courses of study. Such an understanding of prosthetics should be of value in mutual communication and in serving the needs of the patients involved. This can be of the greatest benefit to everyone, particularly in an era when changes in health care funding and management place ever-greater demands on the people in the system for more cooperation and better communication

CHARLES H. PRITHAM, C.P.O.
*President*
*American Board for Certification*
*in Prosthetics and Orthotics, Inc.*

*Coordinator for Education and Research*
*Department of Prosthetics and Orthotics*
*Duke University Medical Center*

# PREFACE

This purpose of this small volume is to provide entry level prosthetists, physical therapists, occupational therapists, physiatrists, orthopaedic surgeons, rehabilitation counselors, medical administrators and others with a basic knowledge of the current state of the art in providing amputees with artificial limbs. The field of prosthetics, like other technical fields, changes through the years, sometimes rapidly, but usually gradually. The information in this book is as current as possible. Trends are noted where applicable, but mention of any current fads have been avoided in order not to risk misleading the reader. References are provided for those who desire to extend their education in the field.

The nomenclature for amputation levels and limb prostheses that has been adopted by the International Standards Organization in recent years is used throughout the text.

Over the past decade it has become fashionable in the U.S. to use the term "residual limb" exclusively in place of "stump," because, it is claimed, patients are repelled by the word "stump." This might be so in the current atmosphere of super sensitivity and "political correctness", but the use of "residual limb" in place of "stump" is ambiguous since the term "residual limb," taken literally, refers to an intact contralateral limb rather than the residual, or remaining, *part* of an amputated limb. A synonym for "stump" would be quite acceptable, provided that it was not awkward to use and did not allow for confusion in communication. It should be noted also that "residual limb" has not been adopted by the International Standards Organization in their effort to develop a nomenclature that is unambiguous, although a serious search was made for an appropriate substitute for "stump."

For these reasons we have made no effort to avoid the use of the word "stump." This book is intended for clinicians, not patients. Clinicians who wish to avoid the use of "stump" in oral communication with patients can partially overcome the problem of ambiguity by pointing to the stump and referring to it as "limb," "leg," "arm," "affected side," or the like.

Many people have supported this endeavor, but I want especially to express my appreciation to Charles Pritham who carefully reviewed the entire manuscript for accuracy and clarity and and made many useful suggestions, and John Michael who helped in the same way with the sections on feet and knees. I am grateful to all of the manufacturers who graciously assisted in the development of the illustrations, and to Michael Payne Thomas for his encouragement and assistance throughout the process.

A.Bennett Wilson, Jr.

# CONTENTS

# A PRIMER ON LIMB PROSTHETICS

# INTRODUCTION

Loss of limb has been a problem as long as man has been in existence. Even some prehistoric individuals must have survived crushing injuries resulting in amputation, and certainly some children were born with deformed limbs, with effect equivalent to amputation. In 1958, the Smithsonian Institution reported the discovery of a skull dating back to about 45,000 years of a person who, it was deduced, must have been an arm amputee because of the way his teeth had been used to compensate for lack of an upper limb. Leg amputees must have compensated partly for loss of function by the use of crude crutches and, in some instances, by the use of a peg leg fashioned from a forked stick or a tree branch

The earliest known record of a prosthesis being used by man is in Herodotus' *History*, written about 480 B.C., in which he reports that a Persian soldier by the name of Hegesistratus escaped from imprisonment in stocks by cutting off part of his foot, and that it was replaced later with a wooden prosthesis. Although the history of the development of amputation surgery and artificial limbs is a fascinating subject, it will not be treated here since it has been covered in detail elsewhere (1,41,60,61) and is readily available to the interested reader.

# THE AMPUTEE

Generally, with proper care, the individual who has lost part or all of a limb can return to a useful and virtually normal life. Amputees can be found in nearly every occupation. This is not to say that every amputee enjoys unlimited opportunity, but when the proper surgical techniques are employed and when the best methods and devices are used in providing the artificial limb, or prosthesis, the amputee without other complicating disabilities can participate in most of his or her previous activities.

The key to successful rehabilitation is in the hands of the surgeon, the physiatrist (doctor of physical medicine and rehabilitation), the therapists, the prosthetist, and often the vocational rehabilitation specialist, but the degree of success is necessarily limited by the characteristics of the amputation stump. Today, every healthy stump, regardless of the level of amputation, can be fitted successfully and, in general, the lower the level of the amputation, the more functional is the stump, and thus, the individual with his prosthesis.

## CAUSES OF AMPUTATION

Amputation may be the result of an accident, or it may be a lifesaving measure to arrest a disease or infection. A small but significant percentage of individuals are born without a limb or limbs or with defective limbs that either require amputation or treatment as if they were true amputees.

### Accidents

In some accidents, part or all of the limb may be removed completely because of the accident itself. In other cases, the limb may be crushed to such an extent that it is impossible to restore blood supply sufficient for healing. Sometimes, broken bones cannot be made to heal, and amputation is necessary. Accidents that cause a disruption in the nervous system and paralysis in a limb may also be cause for amputation, even though the limb itself is not injured. The object of amputation in such a case is to improve function by substituting an artificial limb for a completely useless, though otherwise healthy member. Amputation of paralyzed limbs is not performed very often, but has in some cases, proven to be very beneficial. Accidents involving automobiles, farm machinery, and firearms seem to account for most traumatic amputations. Frostbite, electrical burns, and the misuse of power tools also account for many amputations.

Improved medical and surgical procedures introduced in recent years have resulted in the preservation of many limbs that would have been amputated in earlier times. Newer methods of vessel and nerve suturing make it possible to save limbs that would have had to be amputated some years ago. Highly qualified surgical teams have demonstrated that it is possible to replace a completely severed limb when ideal circumstances are present.

## Disease

Diseases that may make amputation necessary fall into one of three main categories:

1. Vascular, or circulatory, disorders
2. Cancer
3. Infection

The diseases that cause circulatory problems most often are arteriosclerosis, or hardening of the arteries, diabetes mellitus, and Buerger's disease. In these cases, not enough blood is circulated through the limb to permit body cells to replace themselves, and unless the limb or part of it is removed, the patient cannot be expected to live very long. In nearly all of these cases, the leg is affected because it is the member of the body farthest from the heart, and thus the blood pressure in the leg is less than in any other part of the body. Vascular disorders are, of course, much more prevalent among older persons. Considerable research is being undertaken to determine the causes of vascular disorders so that amputation for these reasons may at least be reduced if not eliminated; however, at the present time, vascular disorders are the cause of a large percentage of lower-limb amputations.

In many cases, amputation of part or all of a limb has arrested a malignant or cancerous condition. Cancer is the cause for amputation in many teenage youths.

Since the introduction of antibiotic drugs, infection has been less and less the cause for amputation. Moreover, even though amputation may be necessary, control of the infection may allow the amputation to be performed at a lower level than would otherwise be the case.

### Congenital Amputations and Malformations

"Thalidomide babies," so-called because their mothers had been prescribed the drug Thalidomide during pregnancy which resulted in severely malformed limbs, were born between 1958 and 1961 in Europe and Canada and were given extensive press coverage for many years. However, ingestion of Thalidomide is by no means the sole cause of congenital (at birth) amputation and malformations. Absence of all or part of a limb at birth for no apparent reason is not an uncommon occurrence. Many factors seem to be involved, but what these factors are is not clear. The most frequent case is absence of most of the left forearm, which occurs slightly more often in girls than in boys. However, all sorts of combinations occur, including complete absence of all four limbs. Sometimes, intermediate parts such as the thigh or the upper arm are missing, but the other parts of the extremity are present, usually somewhat malformed. In many cases, amputation is indicated; however, even a weak, malformed part is sometimes worth preserving if sensation is present and the partial member is capable of controlling some part of a prosthesis or even a switch. Studies continue to be conducted to determine the causes of congenital malformation.

## THE AMPUTEE POPULATION

Because of the method of delivery of health services in the United States, it is not practical to conduct a true census of the amputee population. However random polls conducted by the U.S. Public Health

Service indicate that there are about 1.53 amputees per 1,000 population, not including patients in institutions. This rate agrees quite well with the figure in Great Britain of 1.58. If we use a rate of 1.55 and a population figure of 260 million, we arrive at a total of 413,000 in the U.S.

## Levels of Amputation

The most useful method for classifying amputees is by level of amputation. Until a few years ago, the nomenclature was somewhat misleading in that a "below-knee" amputation, for instance, was used to designate only an amputation through the shin and excluded disarticulation through the ankle or amputation through the foot. In an

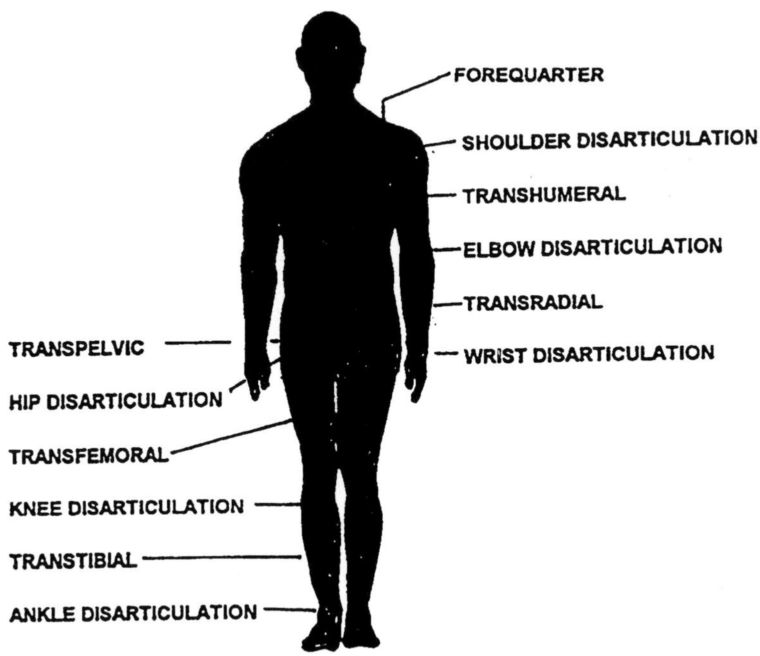


Figure 1. Classification system for site, or level, of amputation as set forth by the International Standards Organization (27, 28).

attempt to purify such nomenclature and develop international standards, the International Standards Organization, through its Technical Committee 168 adopted the classification system (26,27) shown in

Figure 1. Also, the ISO has developed standards for congenital anomalies, most of which receive treatment as if they were true amputees (25).

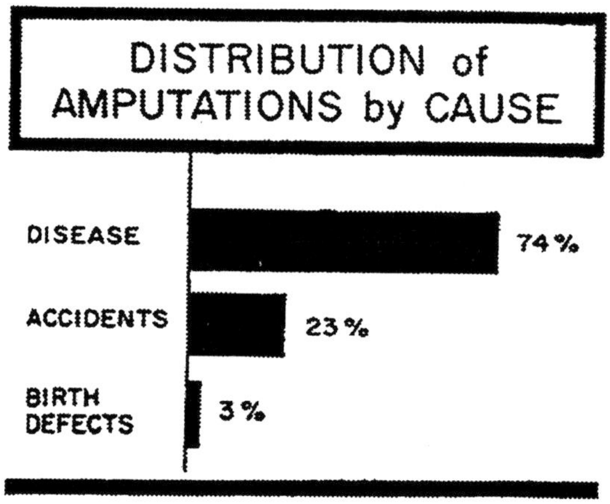


Figure 2. Distribution of amputation by cause

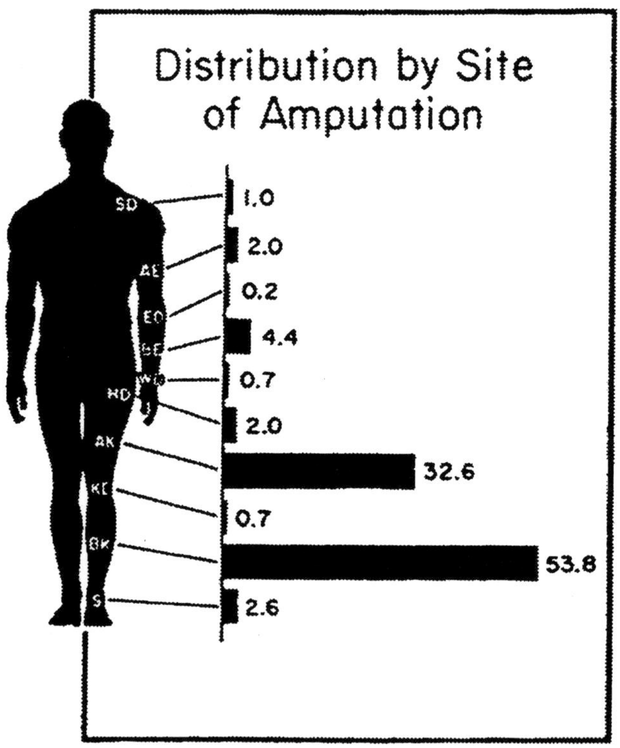


Figure 3. Distribution of amputee by site of amputation.

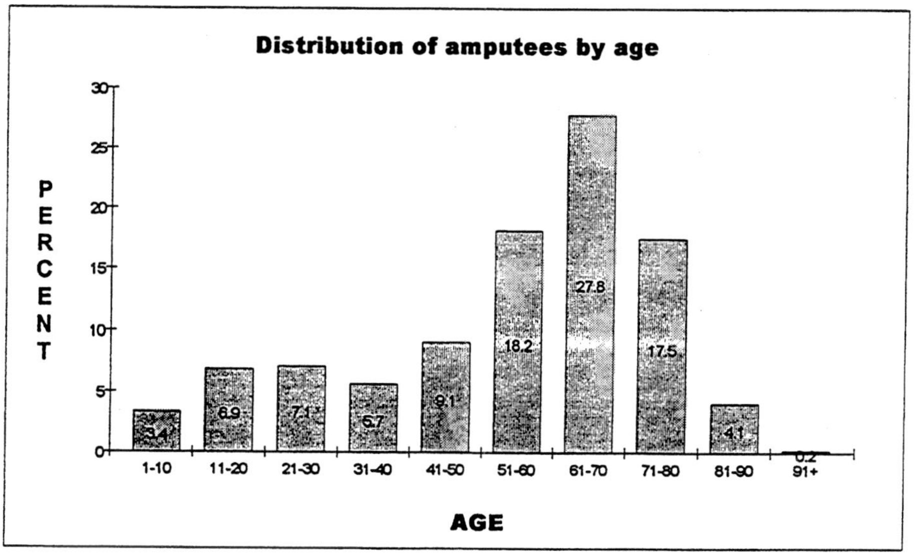


Figure 4. Distribution of amputees by age.

Unfortunately there are no current figures on the distribution of amputees by level, age, and sex, the latest being gathered in 1975. However, there is little reason to believe that the figures have changed to any substantial extent and they are shown in Figures 2, 3, and 4 (30).

## THE REHABILITATION PROCESS

Rehabilitation of amputees can be divided into four major steps:

1. Surgery
2. Immediate Postsurgical Period
3. The Preparatory Prosthesis, including some training
4. The Definitive Prosthesis, including extensive training and instruction

Complicating medical factors and other forms of disability can, of course, cause a disruption in an orderly progression in the rehabilitation process.

For some elderly amputees, the provisional prosthesis may also serve as the definitive prosthesis. For persons of working age, vocational training is often either required or highly desirable.

## Surgery

Ideally, amputations are carried out by surgeons who have a great deal of experience with amputations, but because of the nature of our medical system, the relative infrequency of the need for amputations, and the scattering of our population, very few surgeons have an opportunity to gain a wide experience in the field. Nevertheless, training programs strive to give surgeons the background needed to result in functional stumps. Emphasis is placed on saving as much of the limb as is medically feasible, and to treat the remaining musculature in a manner that will result in maximum function. The use of a rigid dressing is encouraged for prevention of edema and to promote wound healing.

## The Immediate Postsurgical Period

Nearly every amputee feels quite depressed immmediately after the surgery, except possibly those who have suffered intense pain for a period just prior to the amputation. This depresssion is usually replaced early by a will to resume an active life.

The dressing applied by the surgeon is either "rigid," usually made of plaster-of-paris, or "soft," using ordinary cotton bandaging techniques. When a rigid dressing is used, it is left on for 10-14 days, during which time most of the healing has taken place. When the soft dressing is used, elastic bandages are used soon after surgery to reduce the amount of edema and aid circulation. The bandages must be removed and reapplied throughout the day to avoid possible restrictions to blood flow.

Regardless of the type of dressing used, exercises are extremely important to prevent contractures, or shortening of important muscles, which, when present, prevent efficient use of a prosthesis. Positions and actions to be avoided if contractions are to be avoided are shown in Figures 5 and 6.

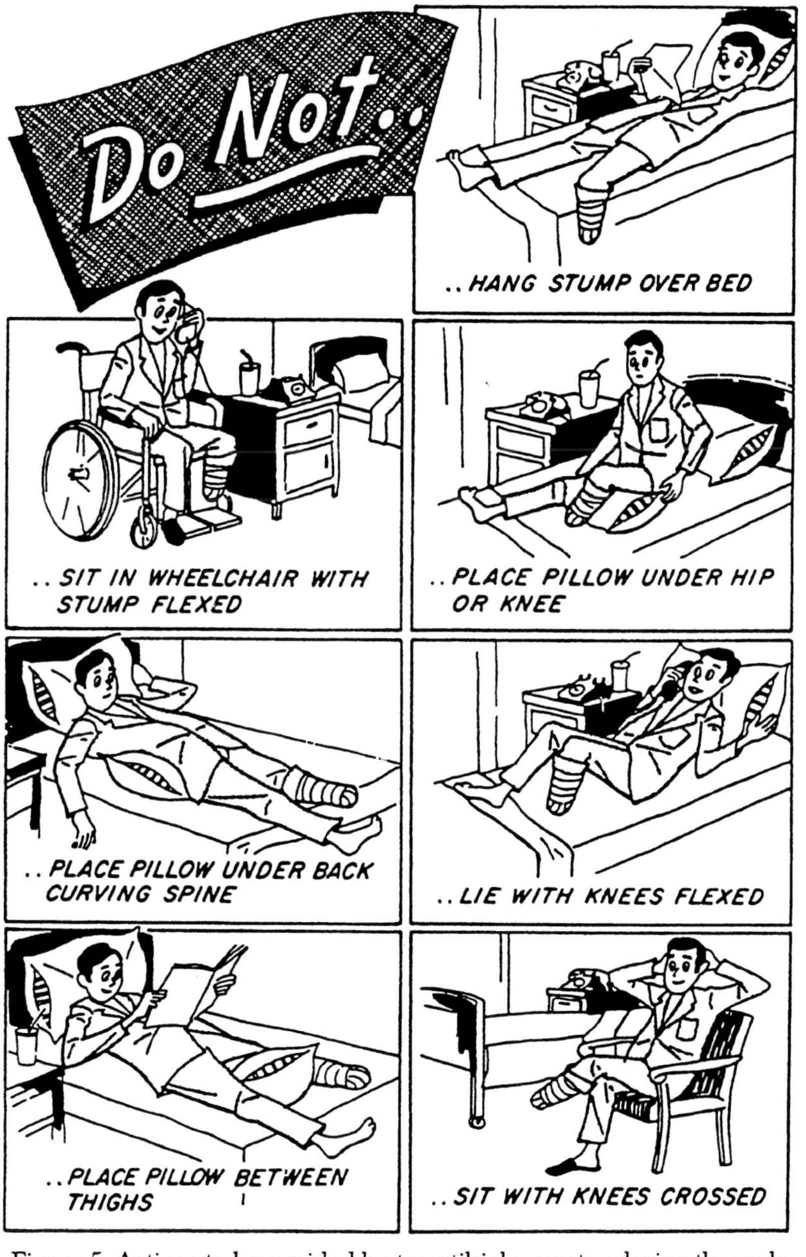


Figure 5. Actions to be avoided by transtibial amputee during the early postoperative phase to avoid the formation of contractures.

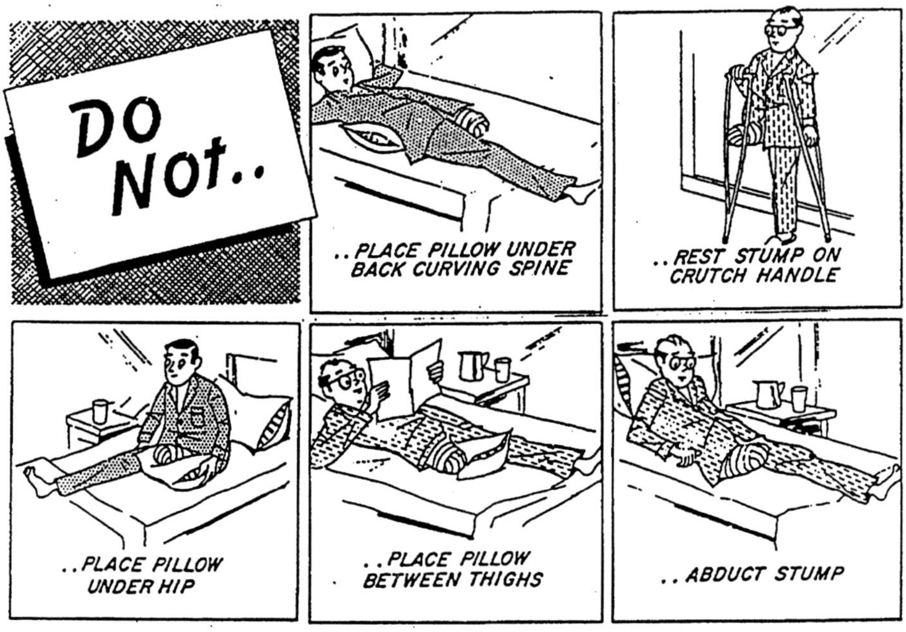
DO Not..
..PLACE PILLOW UNDER BACK CURVING SPINE
..REST STUMP ON CRUTCH HANDLE
..PLACE PILLOW UNDER HIP
..PLACE PILLOW BETWEEN THIGHS
..ABDUCT STUMP

Figure 6. Actions to be avoided by transfemoral amputee during the early postoperative period to avoid the formation of contractures.

## The Preparatory Prosthesis

In general, the earlier that a prosthesis is provided, the better for both psychological and physiological reasons. Although it has been shown that it is feasible to provide amputees who have no other complicating problems with a preparatory prosthesis immediately after surgery, the time involved in providing this service usually seems to outweigh the advantage gained, except in children. The current practice in most areas is to fit a preparatory prosthesis as soon as the wound is healed and edema has been reduced to make fitting at this point worthwhile. The socket of the preparatory prosthesis may be made of plaster-of-paris or plastic and is mounted on an adjustable pylon (Figure 7). Its use encourages the amputee to move about and get some exercise, permits some training to begin, helps in determining the most appropriate definitive prosthesis, and is used until the stump has stabilized.

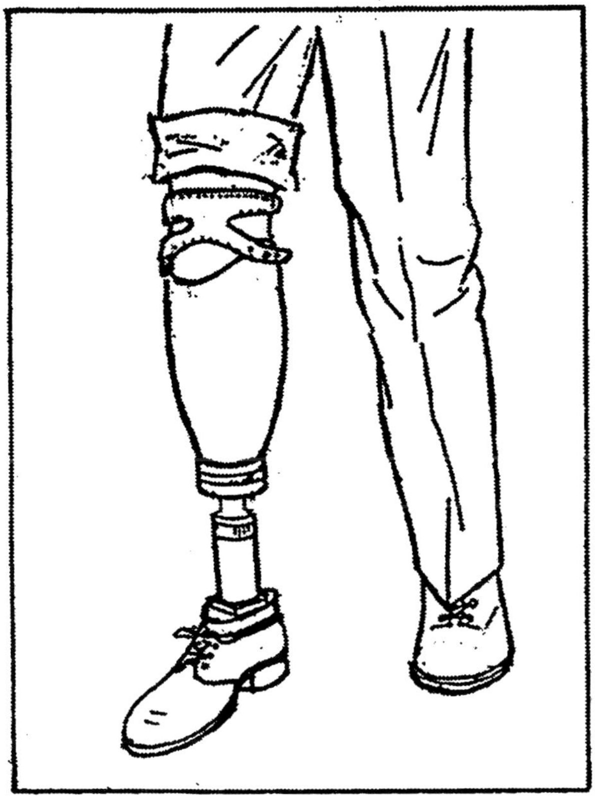

Figure 7. One type of preparatory prosthesis for the transtibial amputee.

## The Definitive Prosthesis

Generally, artificial limbs are fabricated using as a guideline a prescription generated by a knowledgeable clinic team consisting at a minimum of a medical doctor, a prosthetist, and a therapist, and signed by the medical doctor. Ideally, the prosthesis is approved by the clinic team before formal training is begun. The patient and his or her prosthesis are also approved by the team before the patient is discharged from the physical rehabilitation program.

The amount of training required naturally varies widely, depending upon the complexity of the device, the age of the patient, and the presence or absence of other problems. Usually, lower-limb amputees are the responsiblility of a physical therapist and upper-limb patients are trained by occupational therapist.

# THE PROSTHESIS

To be successful, an artificial limb, or prosthesis, must replace some of the important functions lost to amputation, and do so without discomfort to the user. For all but a very few amputees, the appearance, or cosmesis, is very important. It, of course, must be recognized that complete restoration of function at this point in our development of technology is not possible, and compromises must be accepted.

Artificial limbs are made by specially trained professionals called prosthetists, who, working from a prescription, form a socket that provides the connection with the amputee, and to this socket attach mass-produced components such as feet and knee joints to produce a complete artificial limb. Of primary importance is the fit of the socket and the alignment of components with respect to the socket and with respect to each other. The most sophisticated devices can offer very little function when the socket is uncomfortable or the parts are not aligned in a way that permits efficient use. Successful fitting of artificial limbs requires extensive knowledge of anatomy, physiology, and biomechanics, as well as a great deal of skill.

The information presented in *A Primer on Limb Prosthetics* is intended to give the reader a basic knowledge of the devices and techniques available to clinicians in meeting the needs of individual amputees. For more detail on most of the devices the reader is referred to *Atlas of Limb Prosthetics*, a comprehensive text compiled by the American Academy of Orthopaedic Surgeons, edited by John H. Bowker, M.D. and John W. Michael, M.Ed., C.P.O., and published in 1992 by Mosby-Year Book, Inc.

## DELIVERY SYSTEMS FOR ARTIFICIAL LIMBS

Generally, artificial limbs are fabricated using as a guideline a prescription generated by a knowledgeable clinic team consisting at a minimum of a medical doctor, a prosthetist, and a therapist, and signed by a medical doctor. Ideally, the prosthesis is approved by the clinic team before a formal training program is begun. The patient and his or her prosthesis are also approved by the clinic team before the patient is discharged from the rehabilitation program. Most prostheses are paid for by a third party–the Medicare program for elder patients under the Social Security Administration, state-administered Medicaid programs for the indigent, insurance carriers, charities, the Department of Veterans Affairs in the United States, and the state-sponsored vocational rehabilitation programs..

In the 1980s, the Medicare program established a numbering system, or code, for identifying components that make up artificial limbs. Known as "L" codes, this system has been adopted by other third-party payers either formally or informally. To assist in identification and improve communication, the American Orthotic and Prosthetic Association has produced an illustrated compendium (2) that contains an illustration for each unit that has been assigned a code. AOPA provide subscribers with changes that inevitably occur as new devices are approved. The compendium is also available on CD-ROM.

# LOWER-LIMB PROSTHESES

The primary functions of the lower limb are standing and walking. When only one leg is affected, these functions can be replaced to a degree that permits healthy and fairly healthy individuals to resume most of the activities they were accustomed to previously. As a rule, the higher the level of amputation, the more difficult it is to replace function, and the more complex is the prosthesis. An amputee with unaffected knee joints requires an artificial limb that is much simpler than is the case with an amputation through the knee or above. There are available commercially many components for assembly to a socket to produce artificial legs to meet the individual needs of lower-limb amputees at all levels of amputation. The competition in design and manufacture of components is keen, and therefore there is a wide variety of devices in each category and the quality is generally good. An example of some of the options available is shown in Figure 8.

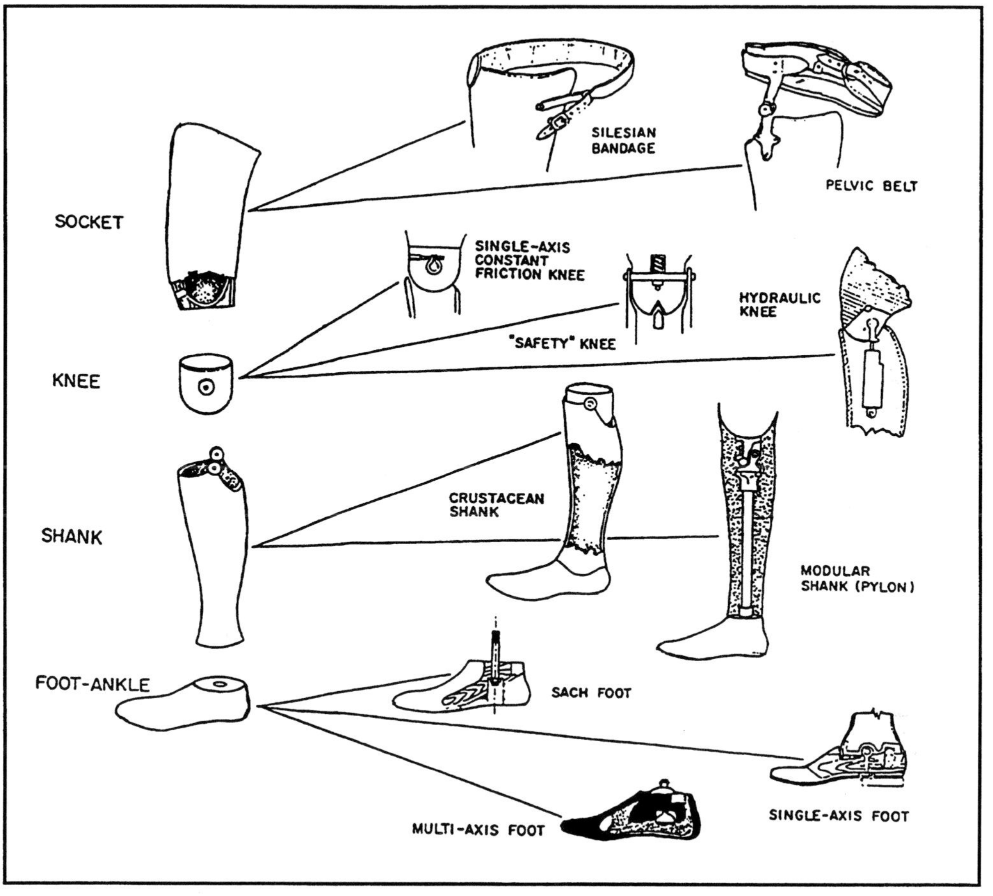


Figure 8. Sketch showing the major elements of a prescription for a prosthesis for a transfemoral amputee. The prescription, of course, is not limited to the components depicted here.

When it is desirable to interchange components, say one foot for another, a special device, the Ferrier Coupler (17), is used.

## NORMAL GAIT

The primary function of the lower limbs is locomotion: that is, movement of the human body from one point to another under its own power. The human legs are admirably suited to provide this function. Saunders et al. (52) identified the six "determinants" of gait that provide for efficient use of energy during normal walking: *hip flexion, knee flexion, motion about the ankle joint* (plantar and dorsiflexion), *subta-*

*lar motion, rotation about the longitudinal axis of the long bones,* and *"double" knee flexion* during the stance phase of walking (Figure 9). The action and interaction of each of these subfunctions contribute to

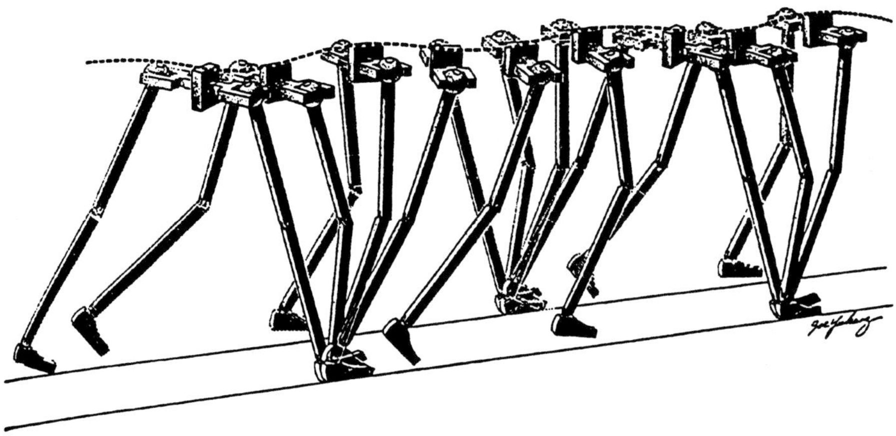

Figure 9. The sum of the effects of the six determinants of gait. The pathway of the center of gravity is a smooth curve in both horizontal and vertical planes. From (52), by permission of *The Journal of Bone and Joint Surgery.*

maintaining the center of gravity of the body close to a straight line between two points and parallel to the walking surface, thus reducing energy requirements for walking to a minimum.

Because of the variations in body structure found in the so-called "normal" population, there are wide variations in the overall appearance of the way individuals walk, but there is a pattern common to all, the gait pattern.

The movement of one limb from the point where the heel of one leg contacts the ground to the point where the heel next contacts the ground can be considered to be one gait cycle (Figure 10). This cycle can be divided into four distinct phases:

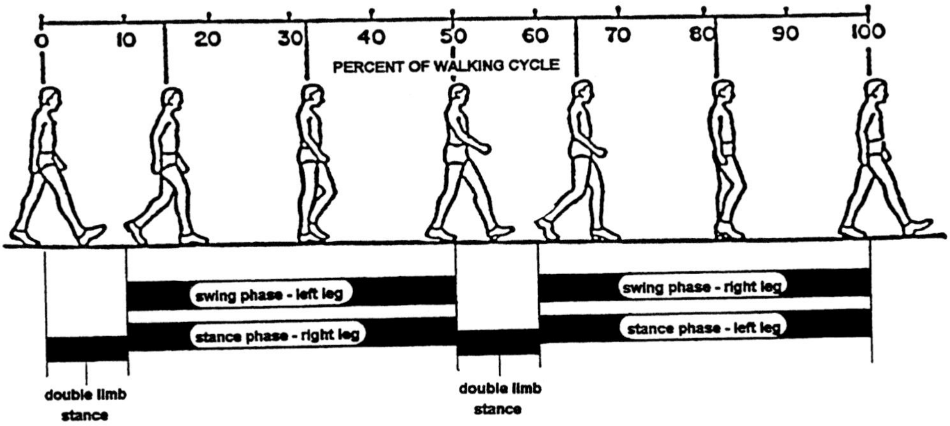


Figure 10. The elements of a single gait-cycle.

1. First Double-Limb Stance Phase
2. First Single-Limb Swing Phase
3. Second Double-Limb Stance Phase
4. Second Single-Limb Swing Phase

The approximate percentage of the cycle each phase consumes is shown in Figure 10. Muscular control of the limb segments about the joints provides for a smooth transition from one phase to the next and is a contributing factor in the efficiency of the system.

The swing phase begins with toe-off. The knee is flexed slightly but sufficient to provide clearance between the toe and the floor as the shank is accelerated forward. Toward the end of the swing phase, the knee begins to extend and the shank is decelerated so that at heel-strike the knee is fully extended. During the first part of the stance phase, the knee is flexed a few degrees to provide a cushioning effect and extended fully again to aid in clearance between the toe and floor of the contralateral leg as it swings through.

When not influenced by outside factors, each individual assumes a walking speed, or cadence, that is the most efficient for him or her (24)(Figure 11). Inman and Ralston (51) called this "the comfortable gait." It, too, varies from individual to individual.

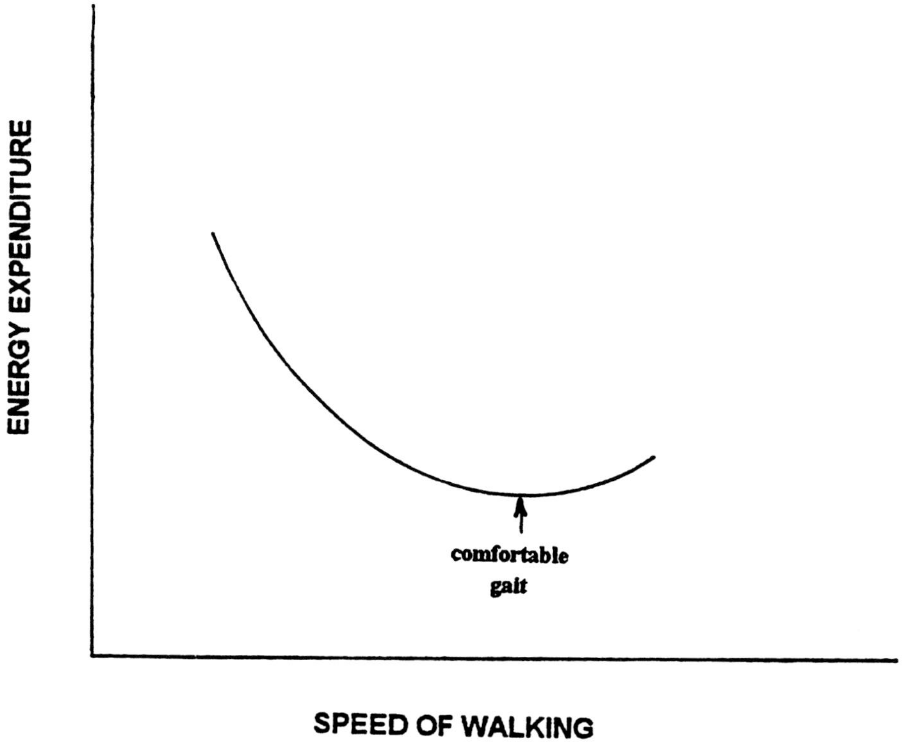


Figure 11. Graphic presentation of "the comfortable gait". A velocity higher or lower than that of the comfortable gait results in an increase in energy expenditure per unit of weight/distance traveled.

**DEFINITIONS**

**Preparatory Prosthesis:** An unfinished functional replacement for an amputated limb, fitted and aligned in accordance with sound biomechanical principles, which is worn for a limited period to accelerate the rehabilitation process.

**Pylon:** A rigid member, usually tubular but not necessarily so, between the socket or knee unit and the foot to provide vertical support

**Rigid Dressing:** A plaster wrap over the stump, usually applied in the operating or recovery room immediately following surgery, for the purpose of controlling edema and pain. It is preferable, but not necessary, that the rigid dressing be shaped in accordance with the basic biomechanical principles of socket design.

**Early Prosthetic Fitting:** A procedure in which a preparatory prosthesis is provided for the amputee immediately after removal of the sutures

**Modular Prosthesis:** An artificial limb assembled from components, usually of the endoskeletal type where the supporting member, or pylon, is covered with a soft foam or other light material shaped and finished to resemble the natural limb

**Definitive, or "Permanent," Prosthesis:** A replacement for a missing limb or part of a limb that meets accepted check-out standards for comfort, fit, alignment, function, appearance, and durability.

## Construction

From a construction standpoint, artificial limbs may be classified as either "endoskeletal" or "exosketal" (Figure 12). "Crustacean" used in prosthetics is a synonym for "exoskeletal," but this type of prosthesis is seldom used today. "Pylon" and "modular" are terms often used instead of "endoskeletal."

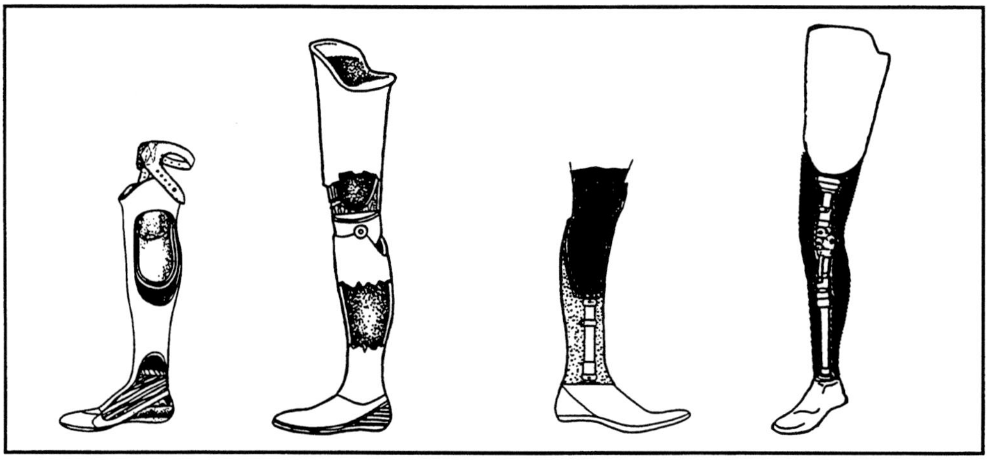

Figure 12. Examples fo the two basic types of construction of artificial limbs. Left, crustacean Right, Endoskeletal. The endoskeletal type is used almost universally but occasionally the crustacean is preferred, usually because of working conditions.

In the endoskeletal prosthesis, all of the external loads–compression, bending, torque, etc.–are taken by a central member, or "pylon," usually a tube, but not always. Cosmesis is provided by covering the pylon with an extremely light elastic foam material shaped to match the contralateral leg and covered by a thin elastic material to provide a lifelike appearance. The filler material is usually a soft plastic foam which absorbs light compressive loads from the side, but more importantly has a "fleshy" feel. The pylon may be rigid, or it may be designed to possess a certain degree of flexibility.

In exoskeletal, or crustacean, construction, all of the loads are taken by the walls of the shank or thigh piece. For many years, nearly all lower-limb prostheses in the U.S. used wood as the major construction material, but crustacean prostheses today usually use plastic laminates or sheet plastic.

Today, the endoskeletal method is used for the vast majority of lower-limb prostheses because the built-in adjustment features found in most designs make fabrication and alignment easier and the cosmesis and "softness" of the leg are appreciated by many users. Still, crustacean designs of either wood or plastic are preferred by some, usually workers in heavy industries and agriculture because the crustacean designs are less susceptible to damage.

As a general rule, the prosthesis should be made as light as possible, a requirement that requires a great deal of ingenuity on the part of the prosthetist as well as the designer of the components so as to avoid unnecessary failures while providing a light prosthesis.

### Components

Feet are common to all lower-limb prostheses and there are available a number of designs that vary from the very simple to the moderately complex. Artificial knee joints for amputations through the knee and above vary from the moderately complex to the very sophisticated. The same conditions more or less apply to the hip joint.

## FABRICATION, FITTING, AND ALIGNMENT

Regardless of the functions provided by the most sophisticated mechanical devices, the most important factors in the usefulness of an artificial leg are fitting of the socket and alignment of the various parts with respect to the patient and to each other. Fitting and alignment are difficult procedures that require a great deal of knowledge and skill on the part of the prosthetist and a great deal of cooperation on the part of the patient. During fitting and alignment of the first prosthesis, it is necessary for the prosthetist to train the amputee in the basic principles of walking. The fit of the socket affects alignment, alignment affects fitting, and both affect comfort and function. Extensive training is carried out later by a physical therapist.

### Fabrication

Sockets for definitive prostheses are invariably formed over a model of the stump, usually of plaster-of-paris, that has been modified by the prosthetist in an effort to distribute the forces between socket and stump in the most comfortable way possible (Figure 13). The conven-

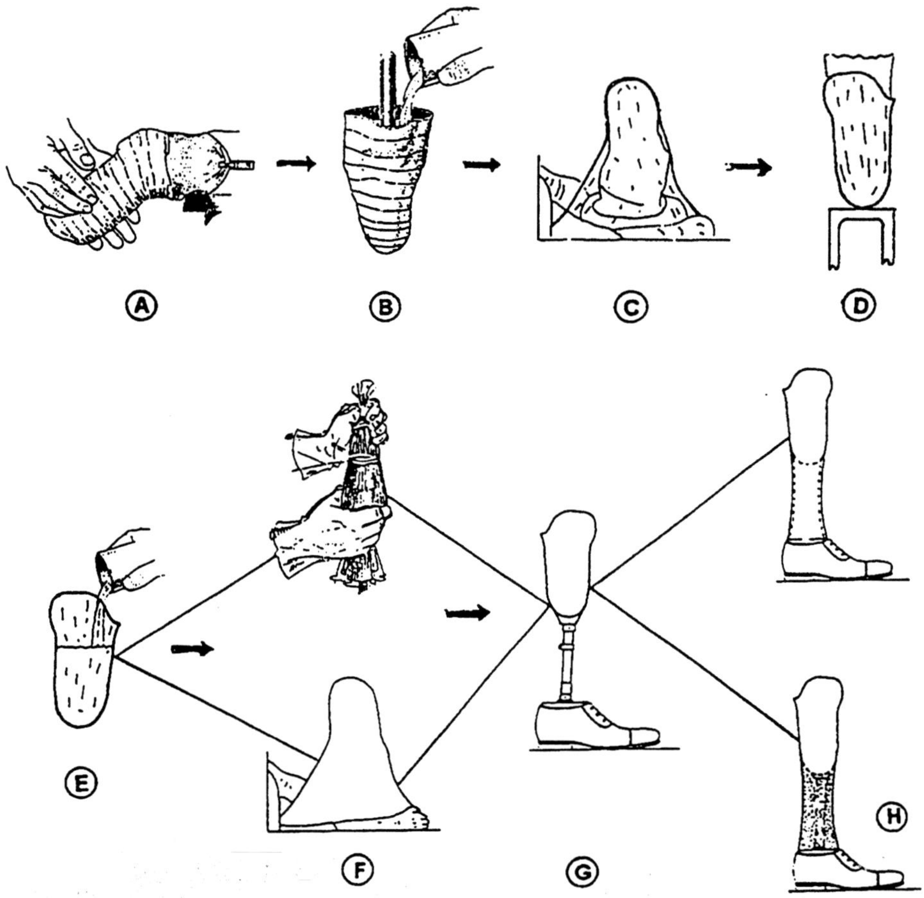


Figure 13. Steps in fabrication of a plastic prosthesis for a transtibial amputee. A. A negative mold is made by wrapping the stump with a wet plaster-of paris bandage. B. A positive model of the stump is made by filling the cast with a mixture of plaster-of-paris and water. C. After modifications have been made to the model to ensure proper distribution of pressures in the socket, a test, or check socket, is made by forming a heated sheet of clear plastic over the model. D. The clear plastic socket is tried on the patient to make sure that it fits properly. E. A new positive model is made by filling the clear socket with a mixture of plaster-of-paris and water. F. The socket to be used on the definitive prosthesis is formed over the new model by either impregnating layers of stockinet with a plastic resin or by forming a heated sheet of plastic over the model. G. The definitive socket is attached to a pylon that can be adjusted for alignment. H. The finished prosthesis may be either endoskeletal or exoskeletal.

tional method consists of wrapping the stump with plaster-of-paris bandage to obtain a negative impression which is filled with a plaster-of-paris slurry to produce a positive model of the stump. When cured, the model is modified by the prosthetist by shaving away plaster in selected areas or even in some cases applying build-ups so that the forces generated during standing and walking will be distributed over the stump so as to provide as much comfort as possible. A socket is formed over the modified model, either by using a fabric and liquid plastic resin or by using a vacuum source to pull a heat-softened plastic sheet snugly against the plaster (Figure 13).

In relatively recent years the use of computer-aided-design (CAD) and computer-aided-manufacture (CAM) have been employed in a significant number of centers in an effort to either reduce the time required to provide a prosthesis or improve the fit of the socket, or both. One definite advantage of the CAD/CAM technique is that the configuration of each socket made can be stored and is available for use in duplicating a socket or in reviewing each case. By "loading" the dimensions of the stump into a computer and using a "mouse" to indicate the modifications required on a model that is turned out of a "blank" of plaster or foam by a numerical controlled milling machine, present CAD/CAM systems eliminate the need for manually modifying a plaster positive model (Figure 14). The ultimate goal is to elimi-

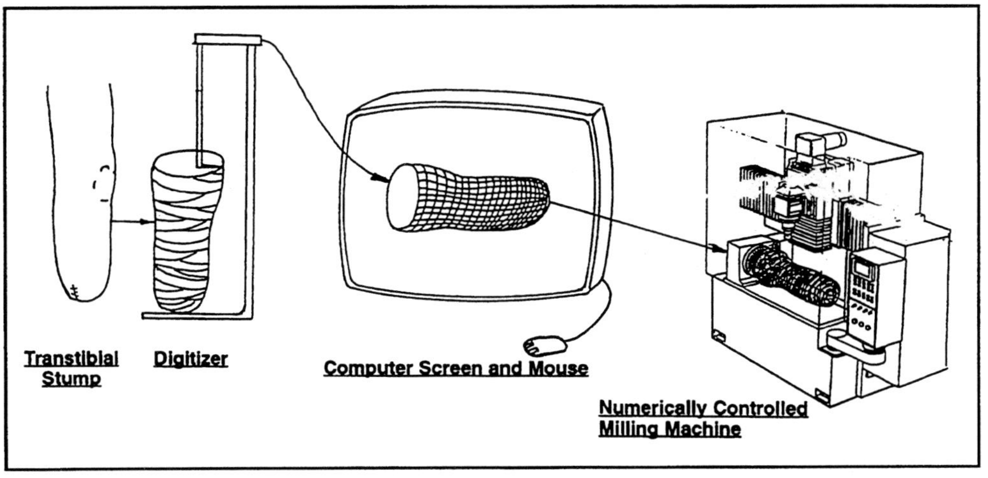


Figure 14. Schematic of process for fabrication of a socket using computer-aided-design and computer-aided-manufacturing techniques. The shape of the stump is "digitized" and the results entered into a personal computer where it is modified by a prosthetist using a "mouse" so that the final product, the socket, will distribute loads properly over the stump. Data from the PC controls a numerically controlled milling machine to guide the carving of a positive model from plaster, foam or some other material suitable for use in forming a socket.

nate entirely the need for plaster or foam. Most applications have been made in the production of prostheses for the transtibial amputee, but the technique is not limited to this level. At this stage of development the advantages are not so clearly defined that every facility has rushed to install a CAD/CAM system, but a significant number of prosthetists have this technique available.

Except in very unusual circumstances the socket contacts the stump over its entire surface and is usually referred to as a "total-contact" socket. The alternative is "partial contact" where the distal end of the stump is not allowed to receive pressure from the socket and may be required when a stump is abnormally sensitive to pressure.

Sockets may be either rigid or "partly flexible" to better accommodate the soft tissues of the stump (Figure 15).

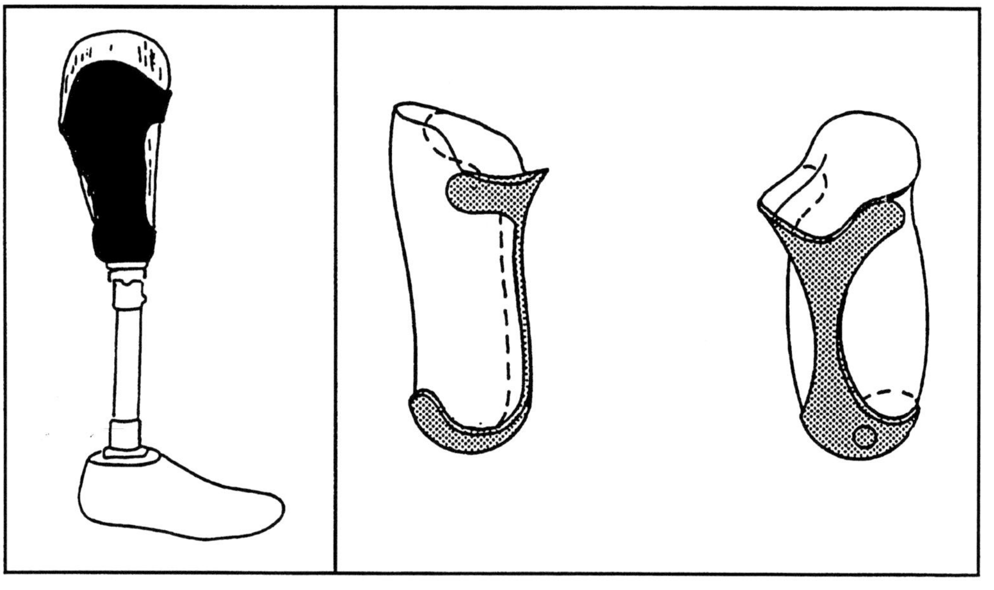

Figure 15. Examples of "flexible" sockets. Left, for the transtibial prosthesis. Right, two views of a socket for a transfemoral prothesis. The flexible inner socket is supported by rigid frames attached to the prosthesis. Illustration on right from ISPO (14) with permission.

Provisions for suspension, which has been classified as either "anatomical" or "pressure differential" (suction) may be incorporated totally within the socket or adequate suspension may require some additional device (Figure 16).

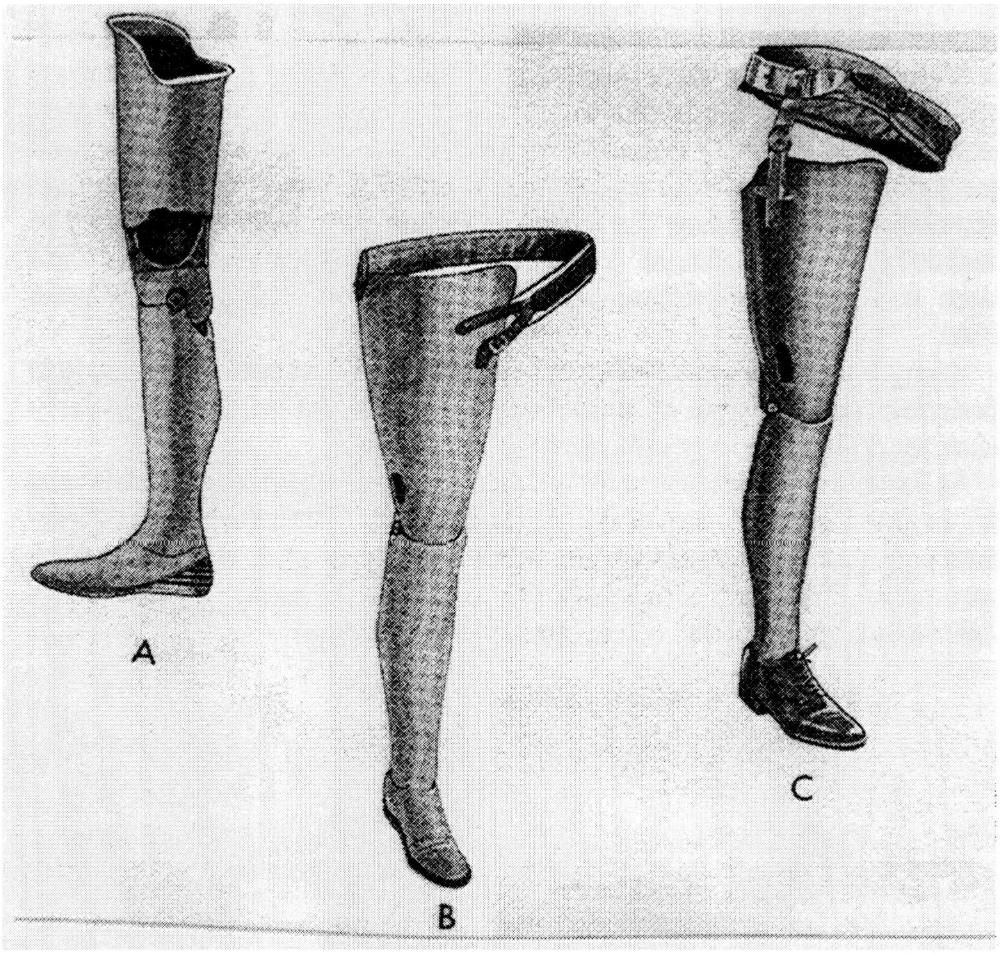


Figure 16. Transfemoral prostheses with different types of suspension. (A) Total contact suction socket. (B) Silesian Bandage. (C) Pelvic belt with "hip joint"– the last resort. Courtesy of *Artificial Limbs.*

## Fitting

Nothing is more critical in the success of an artificial limb than the relationship between the stump and the socket. The socket must fit closely enough to provide a firm connection between stump and prosthesis for effective control of the prosthesis, yet loose enough so as not to restrict circulation. At the same time, the socket must transfer the loads from the ground to the body in a comfortable manner.

Fitting a prosthesis as soon as possible after surgery helps to combat edema. A preparatory prosthesis is frequently used for several weeks or even months until the stump has stabilized before the "permanent," or definitive prosthesis is provided. The socket for the preparatory prosthesis may be made of either plaster-of-paris or a plastic material, preferably one that is transparent. The check socket for a transtibial amputation is attached to an artificial foot by a tube, or pylon, that has provisions for adjusting the position of the foot with respect to the socket in all three planes (Figure 17). For amputations through the knee and above, provisions are made for incorporation of the knee joint.

Because heel height affects the fitting and alignment process, it is desirable that the type of shoe that is expected to be worn regularly after rehabilitation be used from the beginning.

At least one prosthetic sock is worn between the socket and stump to provide for ventilation and general comfort. If stump shrinkage continues, one or more socks can be added to compensate for a moderate amount of shrinkage. Obviously, when additional socks fail to provide the correction properly, a new socket is required.

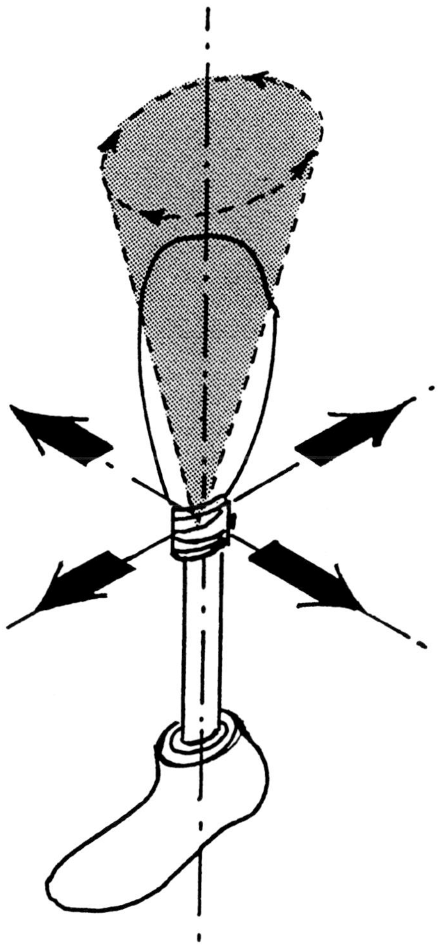

Figure 17. Schematic showing the requirements of devices that permits alignment of a lower-limb prosthesis. (1) Translation in an anterior-posterior dirction. (2) Translation in a medio-lateral plane. (3) Abduction-adduction of the stump. (4) Flexion-extension of the first proximal joint. Length can be changed by using either a longer or shorter tube. Such a system is not limited to a single design. In fact, a very popular system uses a method of coupling the endoskeletal elements that permits achievement of the goals outlined here.

## Alignment

Alignment of the artificial leg is facilitated by the use of mechanical devices that permit the prosthetist to adjust the position of each component of the artificial leg with respect to the stump and with respect to each of the other components in all three planes. These units may be inserted in a provisional prosthesis or in the first stages of fabrication of a definitive prosthesis or the supportive components of the definitive prosthesis may contain an adjustment feature that makes it possible to readjust the alignment at any time during the life of the prosthesis (Figure 17).

## COMPONENTS

### Artificial Feet

For many years, artificial feet have been classified usually as *single-axis, multiaxis*, or *SACH* (solid ankle-cushion heel). However, the introduction of a number of designs, especially with respect to keels, during the last fifteen years, has made this classification system obsolete. A newer classification system is shown in Figure 18. Although the artificial feet, including provision for ankle function, have been relatively

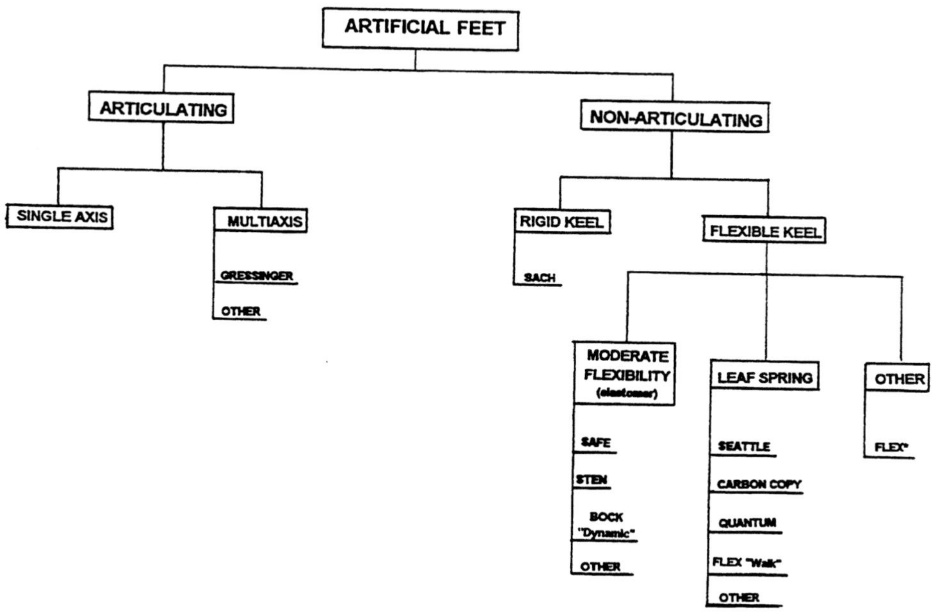


Figure 18. A classification of artificial feet.

satisfactory for some years, there have been introduced to the field a surprisingly large number of new designs, apparently spawned by demands from lower-limb amputee athletes. Many of these newer designs are not restricted to athletes, although the reasons for acceptance are not always measurable.

While the indications for prescription of some of the generic types of feet are fairly clear, it is often difficult to determine exactly which individual design within a class is best for the individual patient. This is partly because certain designs emulate others closely and partly because no one has been able to devise an adequate system for evaluation of artificial feet. The relatively crude approaches to evaluation used so far have revealed few differences in function among the flexible keel designs during walking on smooth level surfaces in a laboratory (4,44,56 ). At this time, performance level expected of the amputee, reliability, availability, amputee and prosthetist preference, and cost are probably the most important reasons for selection of a particular unit.

Described here are typical examples of each category of feet available at this time, and because new designs seem to be introduced often, not all of the designs available are included.

## Articulating Feet

### *Single Axis Feet*

The single-axis foot (Figure 19) provides for plantar and dorsiflexion of the foot about an axis roughly comparable to the normal ankle joint. Resistance to these movements is usually provided by rubber "bumpers" which are available in different degrees of hardness. Some

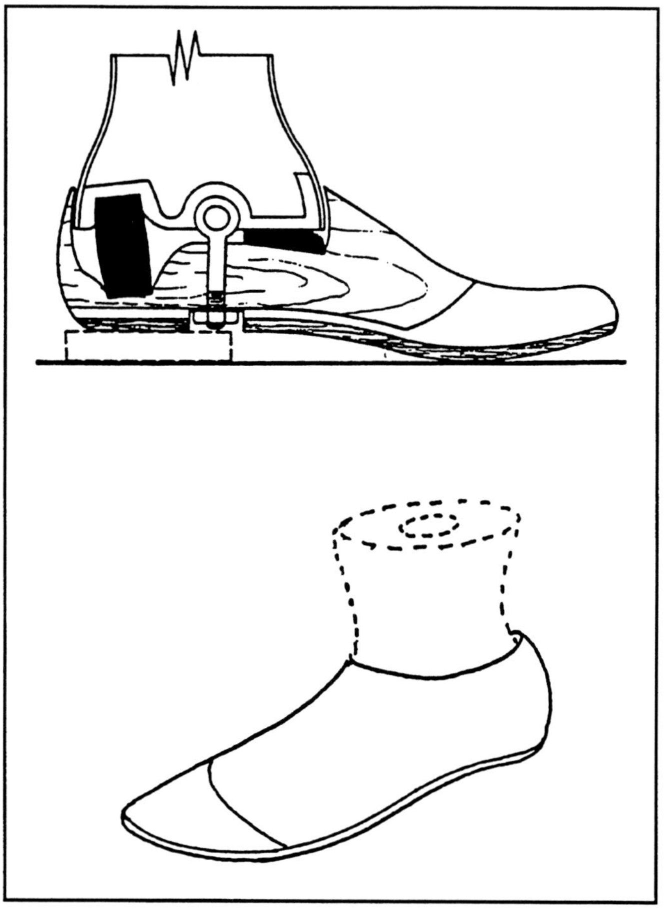

Figure 19. Cross-section and quarter view of a representative single-axis artificial foot. Note the elastic "bumpers" that control dorsiflextion and plantar flexion.

models use only a soft bumper for control of plantar flexion and a hard rubber stop to limit dorsiflexion. The single-axis foot was for many decades the foot of choice, and although the plantar flexion function that it provides permits the achievement of more "alignment" stability, the simplicity, lightweight, and low cost of the SACH foot made it the foot of choice a few years after it was introduced in the late 1950s. The single-axis foot is still available for use when indicated, especially when knee stability is a problem.

### *Multiaxis Feet*

For individuals who are expected to encounter uneven surfaces regularly, such as golfers and farmers, the several designs of a multiaxis foot were used. In most multiaxis designs, a second articulating joint is located in the sagittal plane just below the transverse ankle joint. Its disadvantages are added weight and the need for rigid adherence to a maintenance schedule. The most common articulated multiaxis foot available today is known as the Greissinger foot (Figure 20)(5). Some of the nonarticulating feet also provide some degree of motion about an axis in the saggital plane, and are quite popular for this reason.

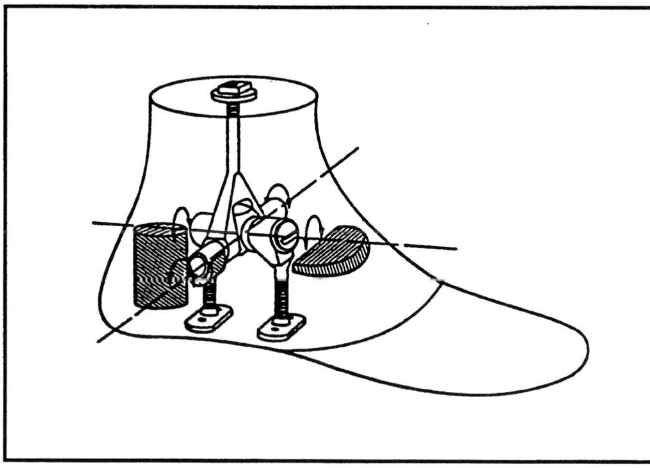

Figure 20. Schematic of a multiaxis foot that permits motion about the anterior-posterior axis as well as plantar and dorsiflexion

## Nonarticulating Feet

### *Rigid Keel Feet*

THE SACH FOOT

The SACH (Solid-Ankle/Cushion Heel) foot was the first design to eliminate the "ankle" joint in relatively recent times even though solid rubber feet seem to have been used with some success in the latter part of the 19th century (35). The SACH foot consists essentially of four major parts, the rigid keel, usually made of wood, the "cushion" heel wedge made of foam rubber, a resilient plastic material covering the

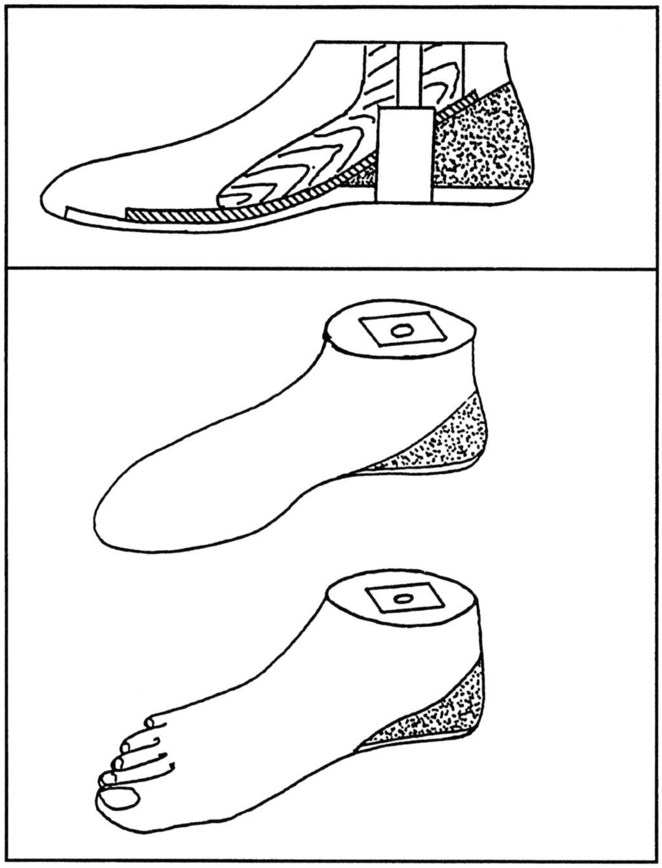

Figure 21. The SACH (Solid Ankle/Cushion Heel) foot. Top, cross-section of the basic SACH foot. Note the rigid keel. Bottom, the SACH foot is available with and without "toes."

forefoot, and a "rubber" sole (Figure 21). The equivalent of ankle function is achieved by the elasticity of the "cushion" heel, and the shape of the rigid keel governs the "roll over" action. Heel wedges are available in three densities: soft, medium, and hard. SACH feet are made by a number of manufacturers, and while the details of design vary somewhat, the principle remains the same. In some respects the SACH foot is a compromise between function on one hand and simplicity, weight, and cost on the other. It is used today generally when a minimum of function is required, i.e., when walking any significant distance is not expected.

### *FEET with a Flexible Keel*

THE SAFE FOOT

The SAFE (Stationary Attachment/Flexible Endoskeletal) Foot (Figure 22)(9) can be considered a second generation SACH foot in

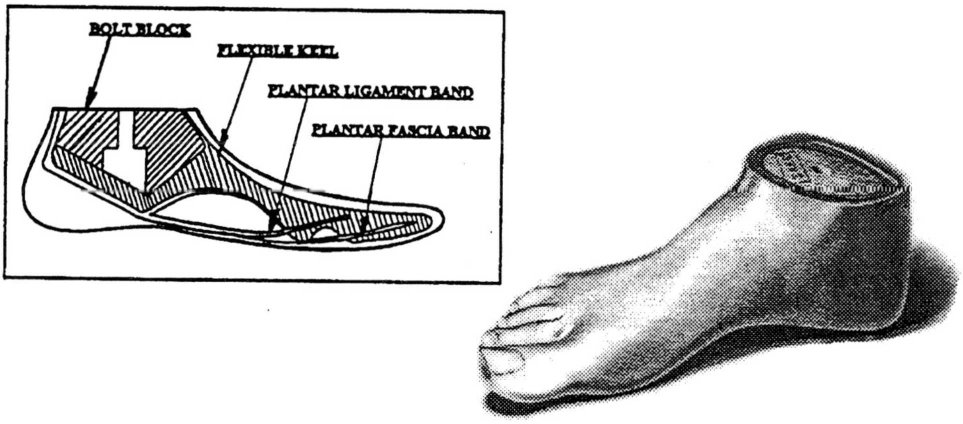


Figure 22. The SAFE (Stationary Attachment/Flexible-Endoskeletal) foot. Left, cross-section of the SAFE foot. Right, the SAFE foot is available with or without "toes" molded in the outer skin. The SAFE foot allows for some medio-lateral motion to accommodate the foot over uneven surfaces. Redrawn, with permission of John Campbell.

that it uses a cushion heel to compensate for the lack of a ankle joint, and the rigid keel and forefoot have been replaced by one with some degree of flexibility, a feature that makes walking easier and more comfortable, particularly on uneven surfaces. The SAFE foot thus provides some of the functions provided by the multiaxis feet without the weight and maintenance penalties found in the articulated models. It could be argued that it should be classified as a multiaxis foot. The SAFE foot is used widely on prostheses for all levels of amputation where average performance is required. Golfers and individuals who need to stand in their daily duties especially appreciate the "three-dimensional" motion allowed.

THE STEN FOOT

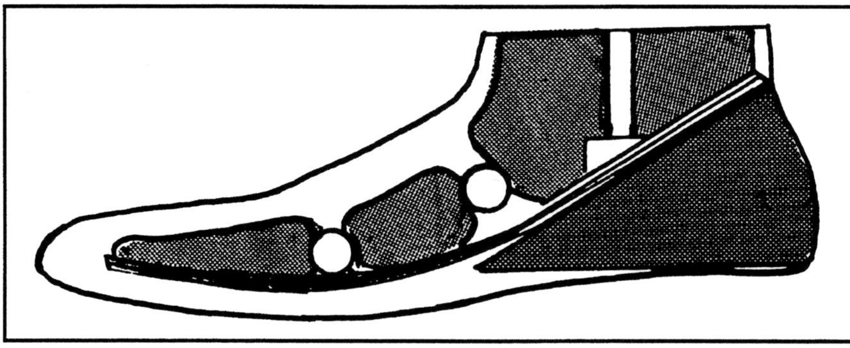

Figure 23. Cross-section of the Sten/Foot. Courtesy of Kinglsley Mfg. Co.

In the STEN foot (31), the rigid keel of the SACH foot has been divided into three parts that are reconnected by two rubber hinges (Figure 23 ). The functions it provides appear to be similar to those provided by the SAFE foot. One appealing reason for use is its availability in a very wide range of sizes and styles.

### *Feet with a Leaf Spring Keel*

THE SEATTLE FOOT

First of the leaf spring feet to be introduced, the Seattle Foot (Figure 24)(8,40) was designed originally to permit healthy amputees to run and engage in active sports such as basketball. Experience with the Seattle foot and other "dynamic response" or "energy storing" feet, as they have been referred to from time to time, has shown them to be well accepted by many amputees who do not participate in active sports but appreciate the "dynamic feel" that this type of foot provides. The keel of the Seattle foot is made of Delrin, a tough plastic with elastic properties that, when given the proper shape, yields during the rollover part of the stance phase and is said to assist in the transition between stance phase and swing phase as it returns to its "resting" position at "toe-off."

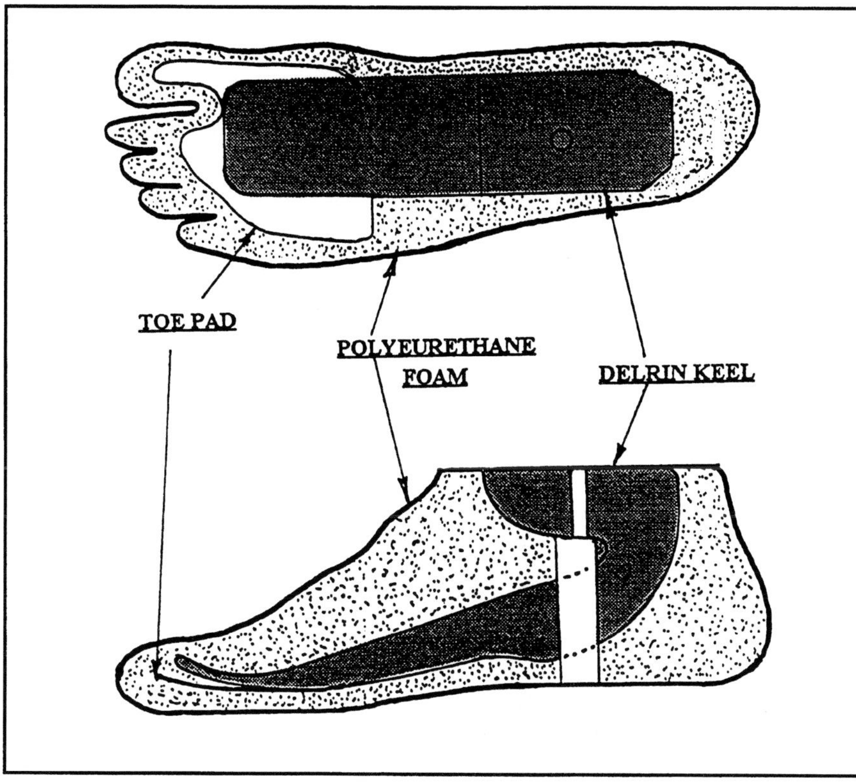


Figure 24. Cross-sections of the Seattle foot. Redrawn with permission of MIND+ (now Seattle Limb Systems).

## THE CARBON COPY II FOOT

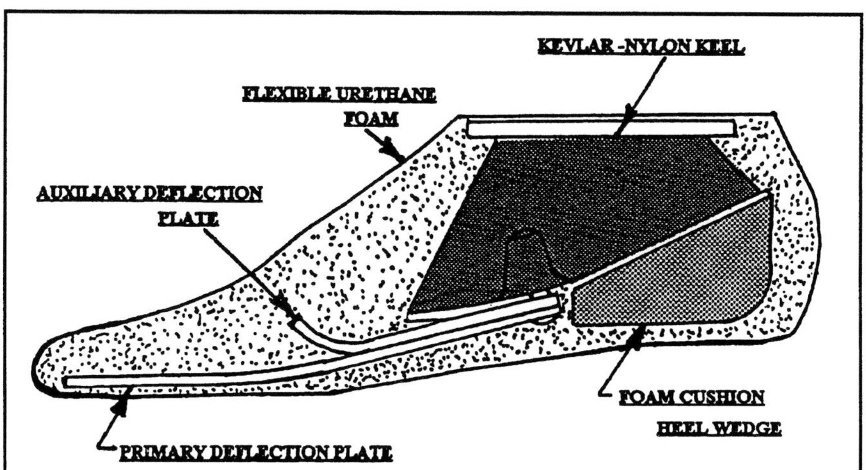


Figure 25. Cross-section of Carbon Copy II Foot. Redrawn with permission of Ohio Willow Wood Co.

The Carbon Copy II (Figure 25)(45) uses a carbon fiber composite for construction of the keel instead of the Delrin used in the Seattle foot, a feature that helps make it lighter than the Seattle foot, even lighter than the SACH foot units generally available.

### *The Flex Foot*

The Flex Foot (Figure 26)(20) is one of the most innovative designs of artificial feet in recent years, in that the keel of the foot and shank

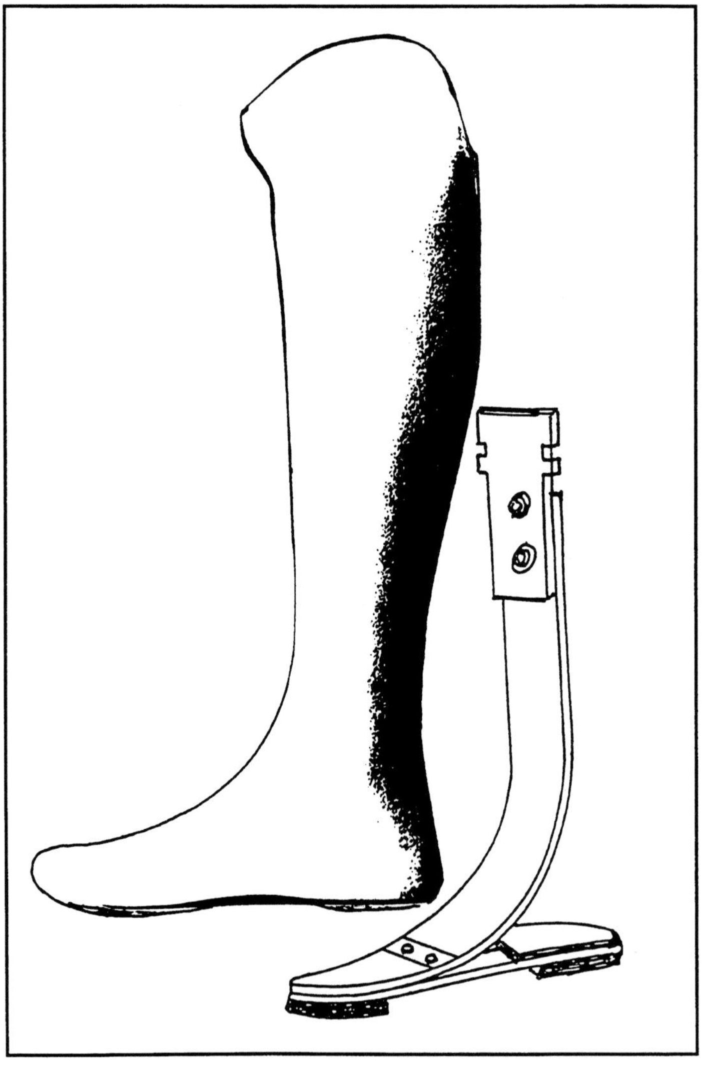

Figure 26. Basic design of the Flex-Foot. This design is also applicable to the transfemoral prosthesis. Variations are available for other levels and special applications. Courtesy of Flex-Foot, Inc.

are formed from a single piece of carbon fiber composite. The goal, of course, is to provide the lower-limb amputee with the ultimate in comfort and function. The original design, introduced in 1982, proved to be popular with very active transtibial and transfemoral amputees. Success with the original design has prompted the design of many variations to meet a number of special requirements of lower-limb amputees at various levels.

## SPECIAL COMPONENTS

### *Transverse Rotation Units*

The locomotion studies at the University of California, Berkeley (16) showed clearly that there is a significant amount of torsional movement along the long axis of the lower limb between the pelvis and the foot structure while standing and walking. Termed transverse rotation, this movement averaged 23 degrees in 12 healthy normal subjects walking at their comfortable gait and rose to 35 degrees as the velocity was increased (16), and many designers have felt that a mechanism to allow for this motion would be beneficial to the lower limb amputee by reducing the shearing action between stump and socket. While the design of such units appears to be simple, the lack of materials with suitable properties delayed the development of reliable devices, but in recent years, several manufacturers have made such units available. However, transverse rotation units (Figure 27), or "axial" rotation units, have not been used widely mostly because some amputees feel that a certain amount of stability is lost, others are bothered by the additional weight, and still others by the possibility of mechanical breakdown and the need for additional maintenance. Exceptions are golfers and workers who must stand at their job during much of the work period.

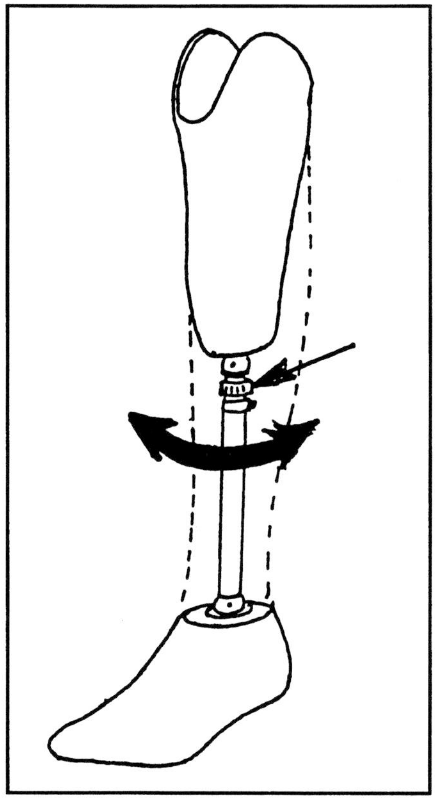

Figure 27. Axial, or transverse, rotation unit. It is shown here installed in a transtibial prothesis, but is equally applicable to transfemoral prostheses to reduce the shearing effect between stump and socket. To minimized the effect of the added weight, the rotation device is mounted as proximally as possible.

## Thigh Rotation Unit

To meet the requirements of people who need or desire to sit cross-legged on the floor or other surfaces, as the custom in some Asiatic countries, at least one manufacturer (46) makes a unit that, when fitted in the thigh structure, allows the part of the prosthesis below to be rotated externally about the long axis (Figure 28).

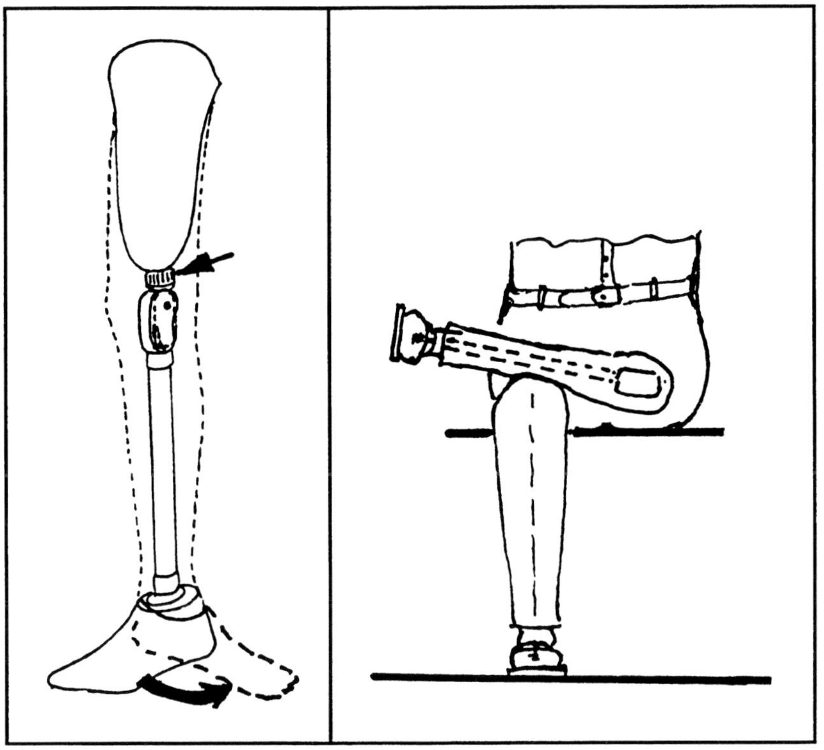

Figure 28. Device fitted in the thigh section of a transfemoral prosthesis to permit sitting cross-legged on the floor or while seated in a more normal position.

## PROSTHESES FOR PARTIAL FOOT AMPUTATIONS

Because the results of amputations through the foot vary so widely, there is no standard method of providing prostheses. Most amputations through the foot, when carried out with attention to detail, leave a stump that is capable of weightbearing, and thus it would appear that provision of a prosthesis would be rather simple. Indeed, in some of the uncomplicated distal cases, simply providing a filler in the toe section of a regular shoe suffices, provided any relative motion that occurs between scar and filler does not result in discomfort or abrasion. However, disruption of the normal architecture of the foot often causes a "splaying" that can make it difficult to use a regular shoe and to achieve a normal appearance.

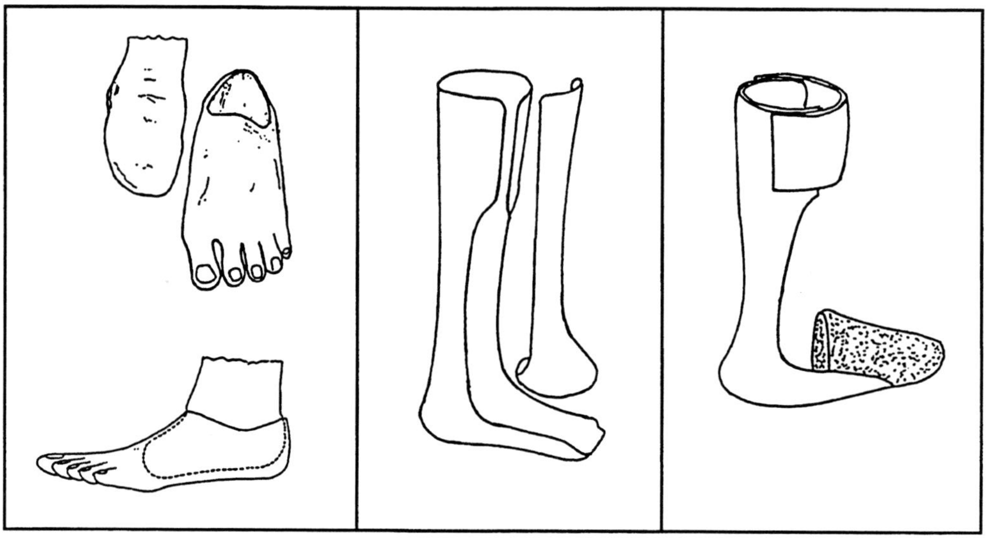

Figure 29. Some solutions to the fitting of partial-foot amputees. Left, molded silicone prosthesis for stump when ankle motion is present. Center, a two-piece flexible plastic socket for use when there is no ankle function present. Right, using a combination of a toe filler and molded plastic orthosis to reduce relative movement between stump and prosthesis

When the stump is so short that relative motion between stump and prosthesis can become a problem, a flexible plastic socket carefully molded to the stump can be used to avoid abrasion and to provide suspension (Figure 29, Left). When ankle function is abnormal or absent a modified plastic orthosis that extends above the ankle joint is usually employed (Figure 29, Center). A toe filler (Figure 29, Right) is used when necessary. Most prosthetists are proficient at devising solutions for the varied problems encountered in partial foot amputations (12). Extreme care must be taken in fabrication and fitting partial foot prostheses to avoid undesirable pressure distribution and relative motion between prosthesis and amputee.

## PROSTHESES FOR TRANSTIBIAL AMPUTATIONS

Prostheses for the transtibial amputation without complications consist of socket, shank, and artificial foot. Suspension can be achieved in several ways. Sockets may be rigid or partly flexible. Construction may be crustacean or endoskeletal. The foot may be selected from the many designs available. The possible useful combinations of features are numerous, as can be seen in the classification scheme for sockets shown in Figure 30.

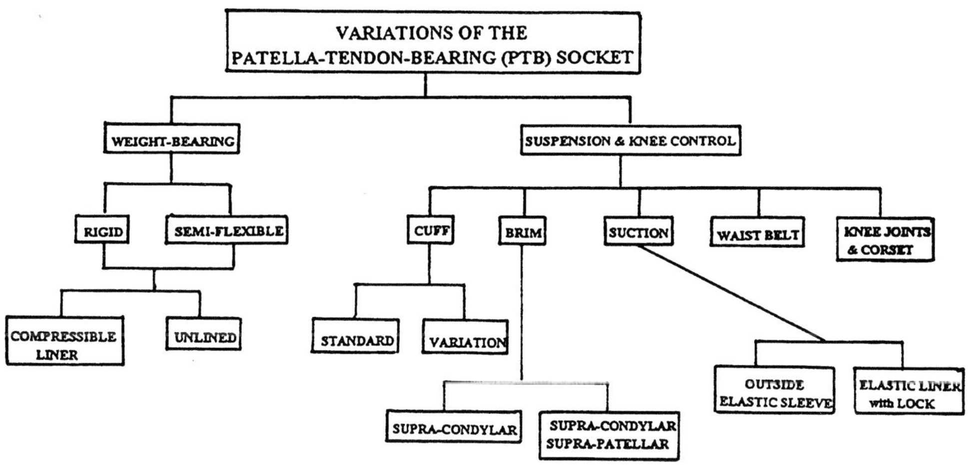


Figure 30. A Classification System for the Patellar-Tendon-Bearing Socket. Not shown here are a number of techniques that have been used in the past but have been superseded by other methods.

## Sockets

The socket, of course, is the critical component in the transtibial prosthesis. For several hundred years the "standard" prosthesis was a socket-shank unit carved from wood to which was attached a foot, usually a single-axis model. The socket was open at the distal end, and a significant portion of the weightbearing load was borne by a leather corset laced about the thigh and connected to the socket-shank by hinged steel bars (Figure 31). As a result of fundamental research conducted at the University of California-Berkeley and San Francisco and the advent of plastic materials, this concept was replaced in the 1960s by a design known as the Patellar-Tendon-Bearing (PTB) prosthesis which eliminated the need for a corset by shifting the entire weightbearing function to a total-contact socket. A soft lining was used and some of the weightbearing load was assumed by the area over the patellar tendon. Suspension was provided by a leather strap around the thigh just above the femoral condyles (Figure 32).

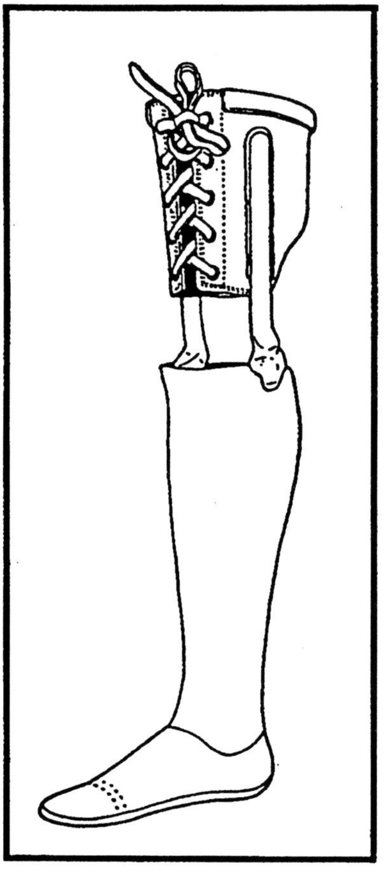

Figure 31. Crustacean type prosthesis using steel sidebars, or joints, and thigh corset to provide some weightbearing. This type was the standard prosthesis for transtibial amputees until the introduction of the Patellar-Tendon-Bearing prosthesis in the early 1960s

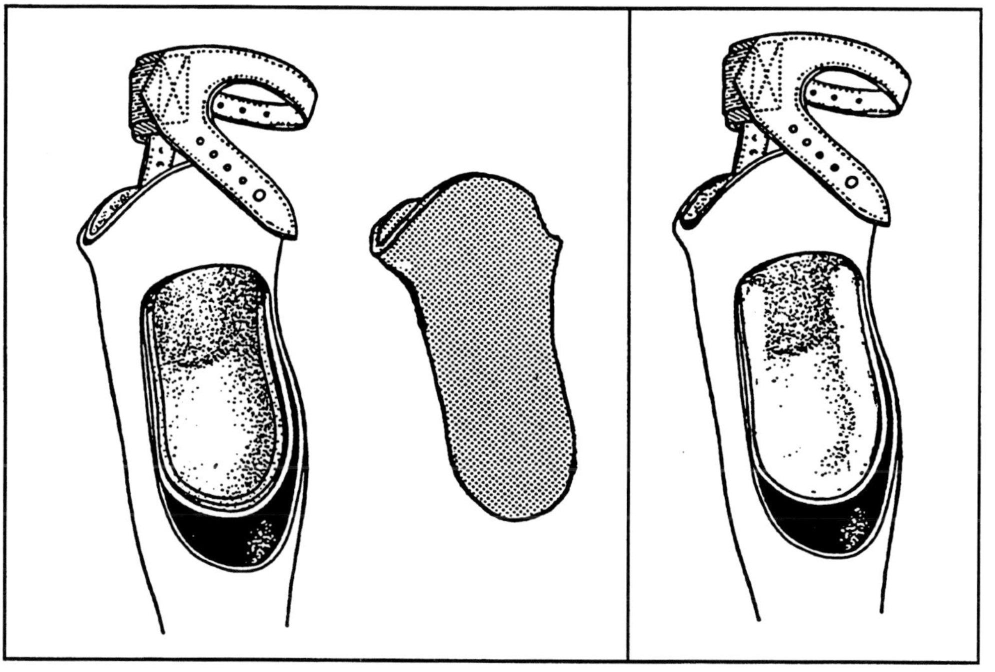

Figure 32. Left, the original Patellar-Tendon-Bearing (PTB) Socket with a compressible (soft) liner. Right, the original PTB socket without a liner (hard socket).

The basic principles of the PTB have stood the test of time, but many refinements have been found to be advantageous, and the prescribing team has many options available in their search for the prosthesis that best meets the need of the individual patient (Figure 30). A description of some of the most prescribed variations follow.

## Socket with Soft Liner

The original design of the PTB included a liner consisting of foam rubber sheeting covered by a thin layer of leather (Figure 32, Left) to provide a cushion that was felt to be necessary if maximum comfort were to be achieved.

## Hard Socket

Problems with perspiration and the resulting deterioration of the original liner prompted some prosthetists to experiment with sockets without a liner (Figure 32, Right). With especial care to detail, it was found that the "hard" socket in many instances was more acceptable than one with a liner, especially in warm, humid climates.

## Suspension

While the supracondylar suspension cuff (Figure 33, Left) can be used successfully by most transtibial amputees, it permits a certain amount of "pistoning" of the stump in the socket and provides no mediolateral stability about the knee joint, a property that might be needed especially with short stumps. Because of the anatomical features of the transtibial stump it has not been possible to maintain a consistent pressure differential between socket and stump necessary to hold the socket in place using the kind of one-way expulsion valve commonly used with the suction socket for transfemoral amputees. To overcome these shortcomings, prosthetists through the years have developed a number of solutions.

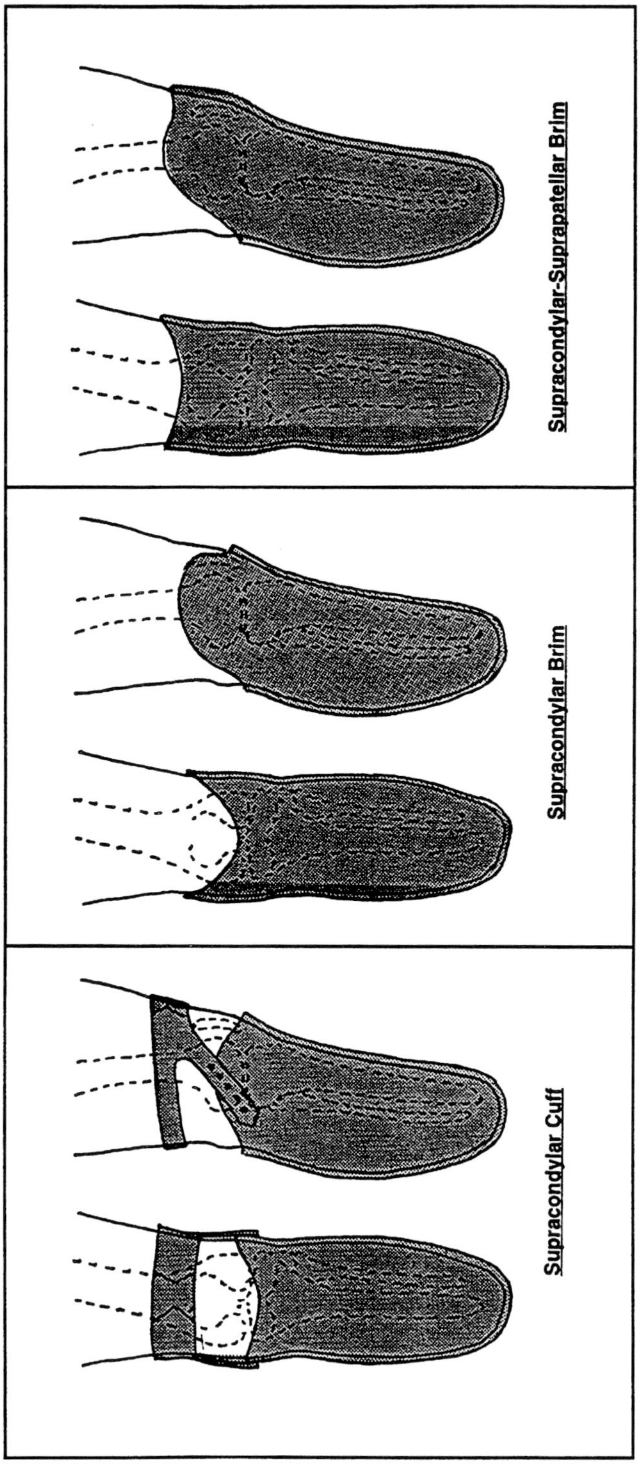


Figure 33. Three common methods of suspension of the transtibial prosthesis

## Supracondylar Brim

In many cases, the need for a supracondylar strap can be eliminated by extending and molding the brim of the socket on the medial and lateral walls to a point above the condyles (Figure 33, Center). In most instances, some flexibility in the brim allows entry of the condyles into the socket without difficulty. Originally, a removable wedge that was incorporated in the brim, usually on the medial side, was used to facilitate entry. The wedge was either a removable insert located between the medial brim and the supracondylar area or it was an extension of the medial brim section that could be removed. This technique could be used if for some reason it was necessary to provide a socket with a rigid brim. The supracondylar brim provides for suspension and a degree of mediolateral stability at the same time.

## Supracondylar-Suprapatella Brim

For those cases where even more stability is required about the knee joint, very short transtibial stumps, for example, the anterior brim may be raised to fully enclose the patella (Figure 33, Right).

## Elastic Sleeve

In spite of the fact that the supracondylar and supracondylar-suprapatella brims provide acceptable suspension for a major portion of the transtibial population, there is present a certain amount of relative motion which is undesirable, especially for the very active user. One way to ameliorate this effect is the use of an elastic sleeve over the knee joint (Figure 34).

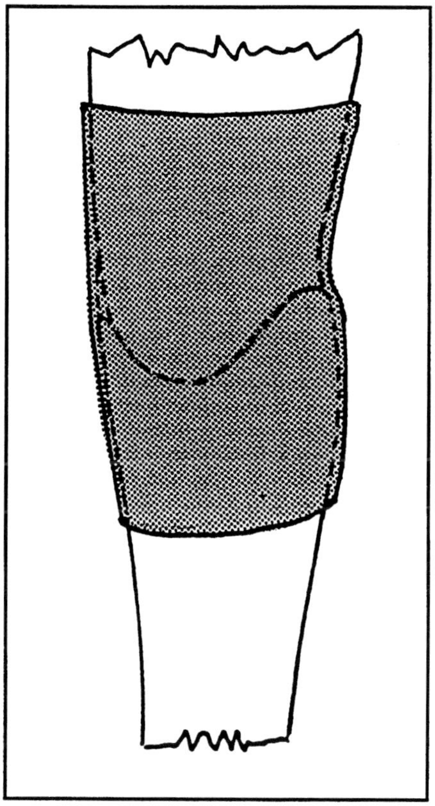

Figure 34. Elastic sleeve for suspension of the transtibial prosthesis.

The elastic sleeve may be made of neoprene, latex, or a comparable material. A series of sizes is available commercially. The elastic sleeve extends from a point about six inches below the proximal brim to two or three inches above the proximal border of the stump sock so as to provide a snug fit between skin on the thigh and the sleeve. An elastic sleeve can be used as the only means of suspension in lieu of the supracondylar strap or some other form of suspension, or it may be used to supplement other means of suspension such as the supracondylar brim when the user participates in sports or other strenuous activity. It is not clear to what extent friction and "suction" play in retention of the prosthesis, but its function is found to be useful to many transtibial amputees.

### *Silicone Liner*

To reduce pistoning action to a minimum, Kristiannson (32) suggested using a flexible liner of silicone rubber that fits the stump snugly but comfortably and could be attached mechanically to a carefully formed outer socket. After considerable development, several very similar methods are now available for general use. Two of these systems, ICE-ROSS (11) and 3-S (18), use prefabricated silicone liners that are rolled onto the stump, and each of the liners are provided with a serrated attachment extending from the distal end that is locked automatically to the socket when inserted into a fitting that is integral with the socket (Figure 35). To doff the prosthesis, the wearer presses a release button located on the medial side of the prosthesis.

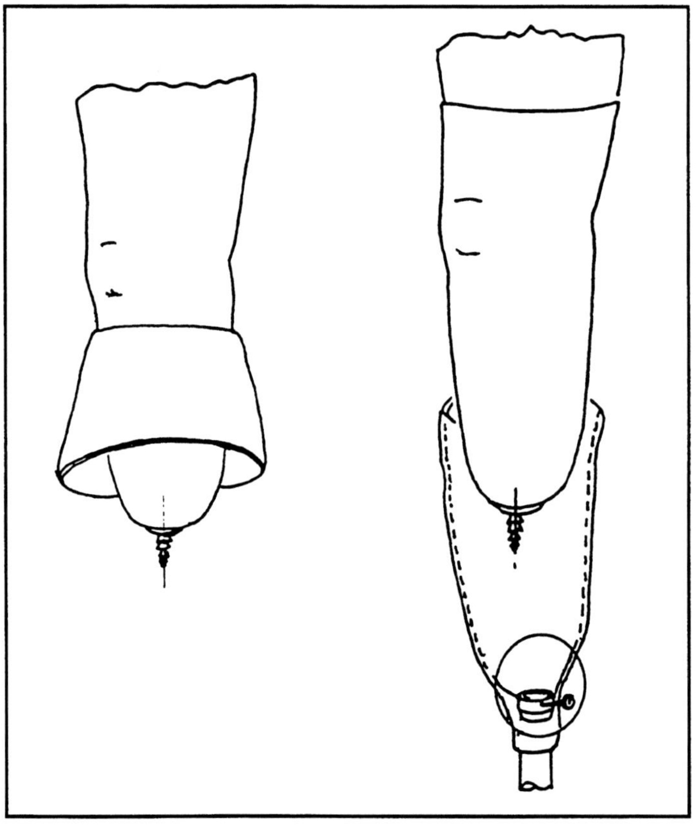

Figure 35. Silicone liner for suspension of the transtibial prosthesis. Left, donning the invaginated silicone liner. Right, inserting the stump and liner into the transtibial socket. Note the control button at distal end of socket.

The silicone liners are designed to provide for attachment to the prosthesis only and do not provide cushioning of the stump against the socket. Their use, however, does not preclude the use of stump socks or a conventional socket liner, or both, when desired. If necessary, silicone liners may be fabricated over a positive model of the stump. Any of the socket brim styles described previously may be used.

Although there have been scattered reports about problems with hygiene and rash, each system has its adherents, and use of a silicone liner as a method of suspension seems to be gaining in popularity.

### *Corset (Thigh Lacer) and Side Joints*

When mediolateral stability about the knee is a serious problem, a corset, or thigh lacer, and rigid hinges (Figure 31) can be used. Among the disadvantages of this method are restriction of motion about the knee and added weight. In addition, extra care must be exercised in the fitting process to reduce the relative motion between stump and prosthesis to a minimum.

### *Waist Belt*

On rare occasions a waist belt might be the answer to suspension problems when conditions of the stump and lower thigh, especially skin conditions, preclude the use of more sophisticated methods.

## PROSTHESES FOR SYME'S AMPUTATION

Prostheses for the uncomplicated Syme amputation follow the principles set forth in the original Canadian design, but fabrication has been made easier by the availability of feet modified especially for use with the long stump. To improve the strength of the original design, the two-piece construction has been replaced by either a window in the narrow portion of the socket or an elastic foam insert in this area of a more cylindrical socket (Figure 36). Provisions for additional or alternative methods of suspension are rarely, if ever, required. When the stump is not capable of full weightbearing, the socket can be extended proximally and shaped so any portion of the weightbearing load can be transferred to the flares of the tibial condyles as desired.

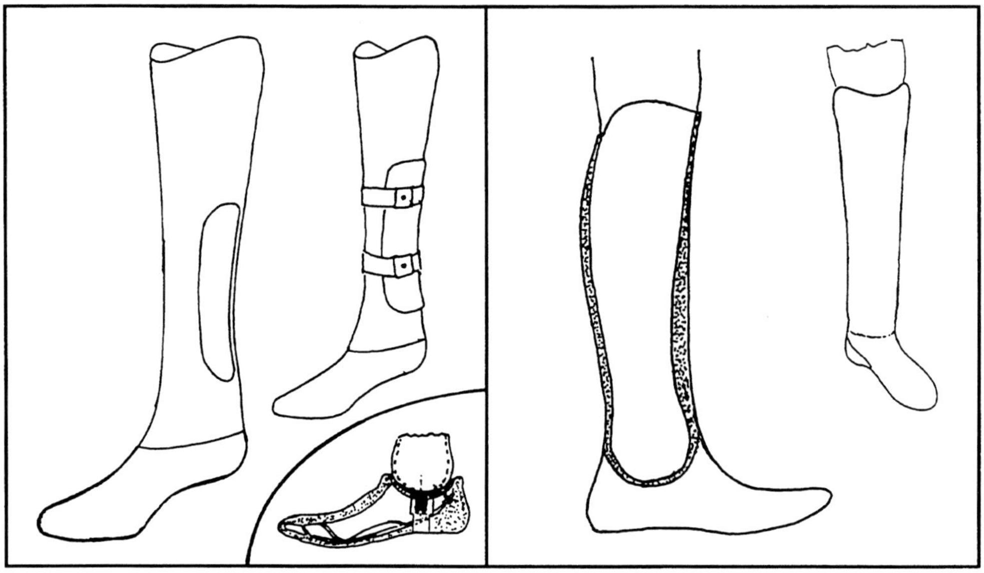

Figure 36. Two methods of fitting prostheses for Syme's amputation or ankle disarticulation. Left, Use of cutout, or window, on medial wall to permit passage of bulbous stump. Cross-section of a foot designed especially for the Syme stump is shown in the inset. Right, "cylindrical" socket lined with an elastic foam to permit passage of the bulbous stump. This arrangement also provides suspension for the prosthesis.

Feet designed for use by the Syme amputee are inherently somewhat weaker than those designed for higher levels, a fact that should be recognized by all concerned.

## PROSTHESES FOR TRANSFEMORAL AMPUTATIONS

A typical prosthesis for the transfemoral amputee is composed of four basic components: the *socket*, the *knee system*, the *shank*, and the *foot-ankle system* (Figure 37). When "suction" is not a feasible means for retaining the socket in place, an alternate *suspension system* is required. A wide variety of knee units, shanks, and feet is available from a number of manufacturers for use in assembling a prosthesis to meet the individual needs of transfemoral amputees. Fortunately, most of the devices of each manufacturer are interchangeable with devices of other manufacturers and many can be used with either endoskeletal or exoskeletal construction, thus providing the clinical team with a wide range of options in preparing prescriptions.

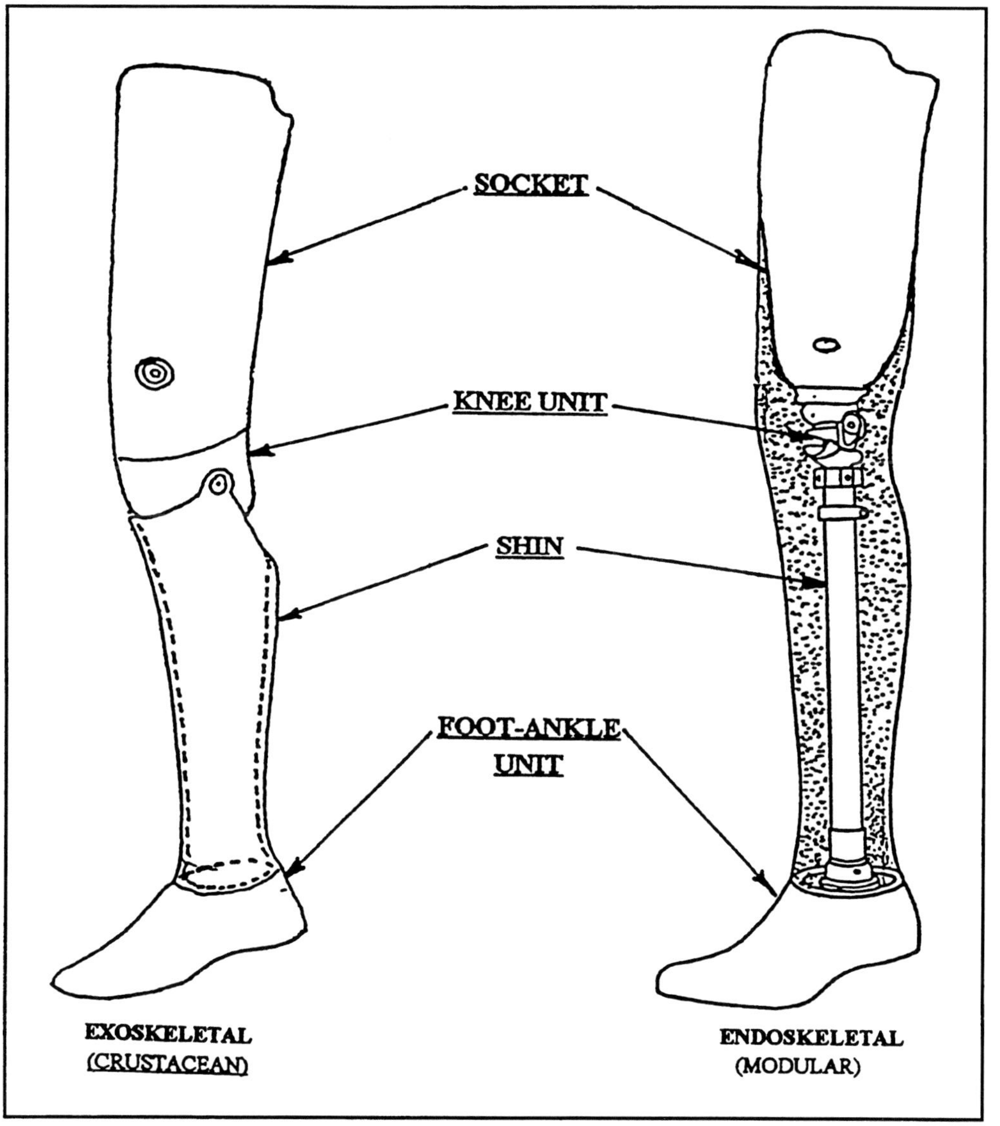


Figure 37. Two basic types of construction for transfemoral amputees. Left, exoskeleton, or crustacean, where the stresses from weight-bearing are carried in the outer wall of the shin. Right, Endoskeletal, sometimes referred to as "plyon" and modular, where the stresses are carried by a central strut, usually tubular. The shape of the leg is usually obtained by using a resilient foam under a flexible plastic cosmetic cover. The endoskeletal type is by far the most popular type in use at this time.

## Sockets

Two closely related socket designs are in use in the U.S. today as a result of experience with the original "quadrilateral" socket developed at the University of California, Berkeley in the late 1940s: the "total contact quadrilateral" socket and the "ischial containment" socket (Figure 38). The total contact quadrilateral socket was used universally until the mid 1980s when a small group of prosthetists began experiments designed to enhance the comfort of the transfemoral amputee.

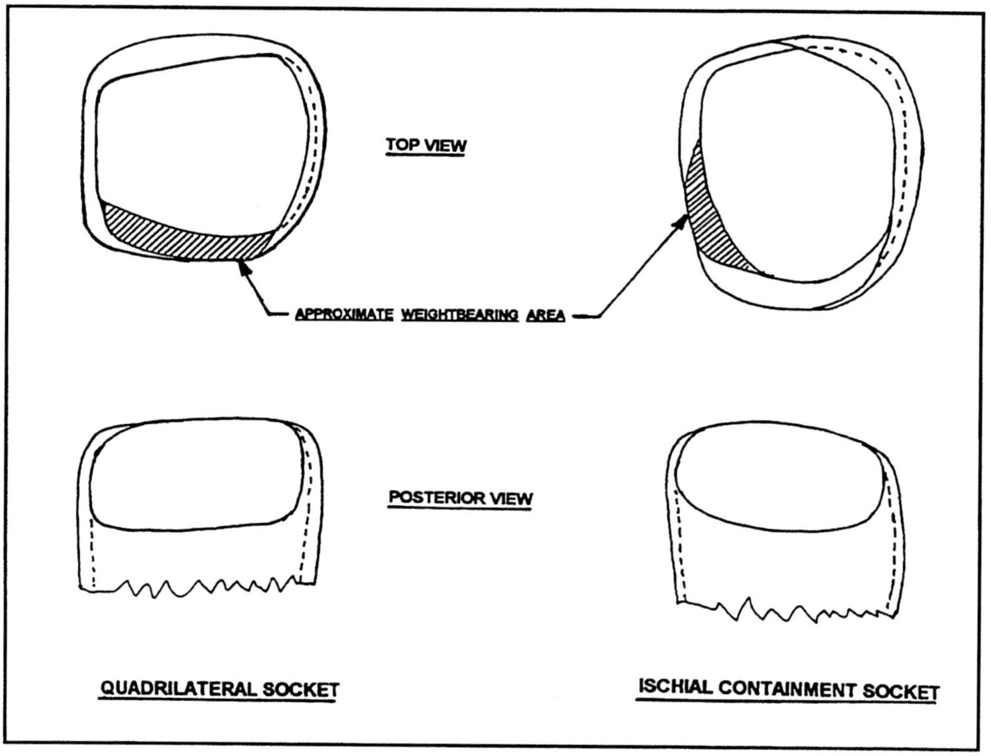


Figure 38. Schematic of socket brims to show some of the differences between the "quadrilateral" and "ischial containment" sockets for transfemoral amputees. Many sockets in clinical practice combine features of both designs.

The result was touted as an entirely new approach to management of the transfemoral amputee, but a close examination revealed that the two designs had more in common than differences (14). The lines between the two designs are a bit blurred, the main difference being that the posterior brim of the ischial containment version encompasses more of the stump in a slightly different configuration of the quadrilateral socket. Both sockets are used today, the preference generally being left to the prosthetist, and the result is often a compromise between the two designs.

## Suspension Systems

The most common suspension system for the active user of transfemoral prostheses is the "suction" socket where a one-way expulsion valve is located at the distal portion of the socket to provide a pressure differential between stump and socket (Figure 39). The suction socket provides the maximum amount of freedom possible for control of

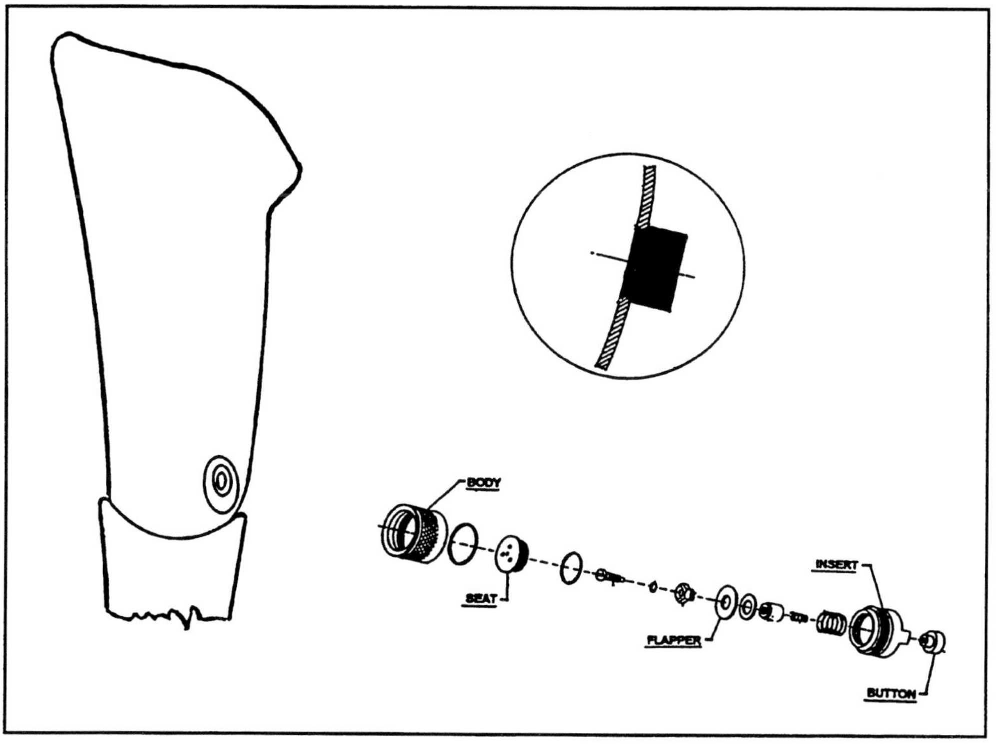


Figure 39. Schematic of suction socket valve and a commonly used location for it.

the prosthesis. Because no sock is worn between the stump and socket, a few users encounter a skin reaction, and some other method of suspension is required.

A certain amount of strength and balance is needed for donning the prosthesis, a requirement that can be excessive for some older patients. In these cases, the socket may be fitted a bit looser and a prosthetic sock is used in conjunction with a Silesian Bandage (Figure 40, Left), a device designed and located so that freedom of motion is restricted only marginally and is often recommended for use with a "suction" valve when there might be a danger of losing suction. A

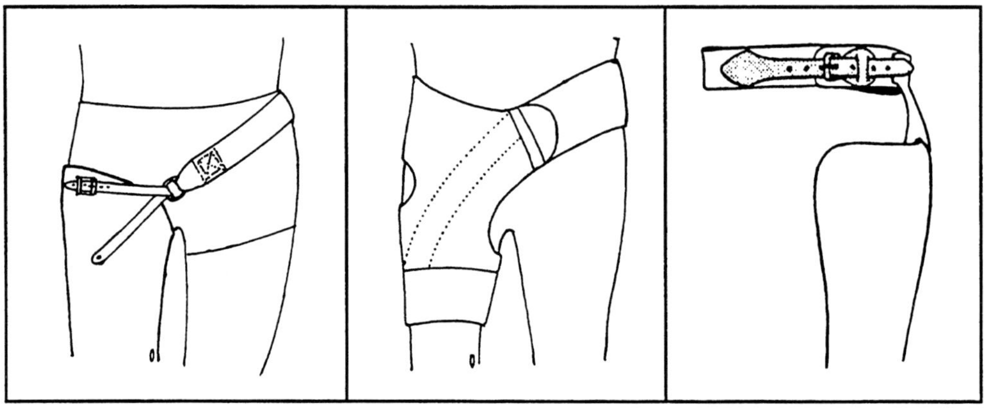

Figure 40. Some methods of suspension for transfemoral protheses. Left, silesian bandage; center, TES belt (Total Elastic Suspension); right, pelvic belt. The silesian bandage and the TES belt are used with a suction socket when suction is difficult to maintain constantly. The pelvic belt is restrictive and is used as a last resort

recent innovation which seems to be used at an increasing rate for suspension of the transfemoral prosthesis is the TES (Total Elastic Auxiliary Suspension) Belt (Figure 40, Center), which is an elastic system that conforms closely to the torso. Velcro is used to permit easy adjustability. When the Silesian Bandage or the TES Belt are contraindicated a pelvic belt with "hip" joint is used (Figure 40, Right). This technique is restrictive and is considered to be the last resort for suspension of the transfemoral prosthesis.

Experiments have shown that the use of a flexible silicone liner as an inner socket that can be attached mechanically to an outer socket in the same manner that is being used successfully for transtibial amputees is probably practical, but as yet such a system has not found its way into general practice.

## Flexible-Wall Sockets

For many years, it has been recognized that sockets with flexible walls and brims would be more comfortable than those with rigid brims, but attempts to achieve a durable socket of this design were unsuccessful until the availability of flexible plastics such as polypropylene, polyethylene, and Surlyn, which permitted relatively easy fabrication because they could be formed easily over a plaster-of-paris cast when heated to about 400 deg. F. However, while the durability of sockets made of these materials early in the development phase outlasted the results of previous efforts, cost-effectiveness was

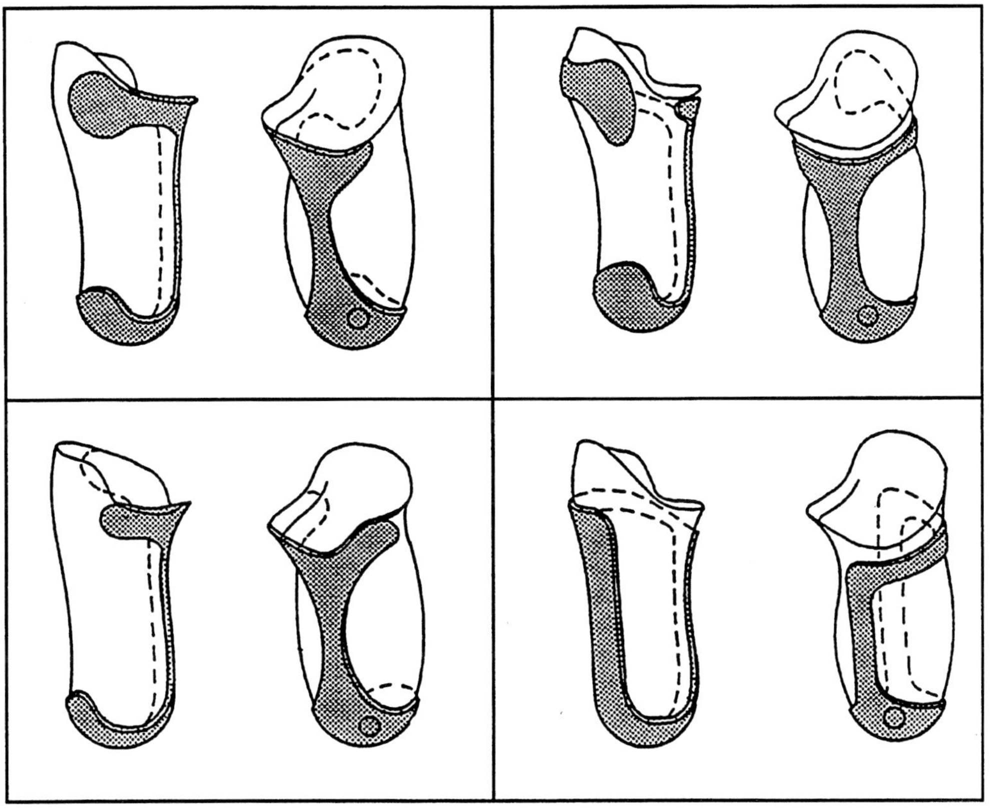

Figure 41. Four different designs of rigid frames for supporting a flexible socket. From ISPO (14) with permission.

marginal until recently when better materials have become available. Present designs (Figure 41) consist of a flexible socket formed from sheet plastic over a carefully modified cast and supported by a rigid frame that is attached to the knee unit.

The flexible-wall socket designs may be used with either the quadrilateral or the ischial containment configuration, though the design of the rigid frame may vary. There seems to be no doubt that the flexible socket affords more comfort, the only drawback probably being an increase in cost.

## Knee Units

To permit the transfemoral amputee to be seated comfortably might be considered the first reason for using a joint that can be flexed. At the same time, such a joint makes it possible for the transfemoral amputee to walk with a gait that approaches a normal pattern. When the shank of an artificial leg is allowed to swing freely about the knee joint, the amputee is restricted to walking slowly, using short steps, but there are several methods available to make walking easier, more efficient, and with a more natural motion and thus a more natural appearance.

As a result of research, development, and competition among manufacturers, there is a myriad of artificial knee units available to meet the needs of all types of transfemoral amputees, whether sedentary, moderately active, or extremely active. Aside from providing stable support during standing and the ability to flex for sitting, the artificial knee has two major and distinct functions: *control of the shank during the swing phase of walking* and *control of the knee during standing and the stance phase of walking.* These functions may be independent of each other or they may be interdependent. As a result, classification of knee units is not an easy task. A rather simplified approach is shown in Figure 42.

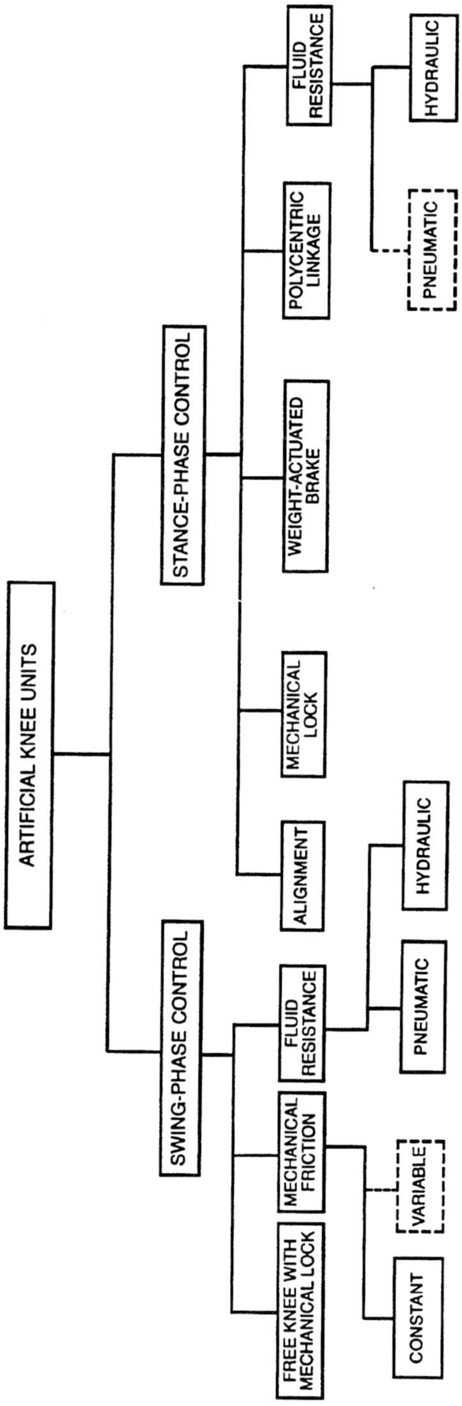


Figure 42. A classification system for artificial knee units. Units presented by boxes with broken lines are not available

## Swing-Phase Control

One way to control action of the shank during walking is to simply lock the knee, and knee units that will lock automatically upon full extension are available for patients who are feeble or otherwise unable to control a knee as it flexes and extends during walking. Of course, walking with a knee locked in the extended position requires either an abducted swing or vaulting, which is ungainly while requiring a significant amount of unnecessary energy. Shortening the prosthesis slightly improves toe clearance but causes the user to "step into a hole" as he walks.

When the shank of an artificial leg is allowed to swing freely about the knee joint, the amputee is restricted to walking slowly using very short steps. The simplest way to permit faster gait safely is to introduce a certain amount of friction into the joint to keep the shank from swinging back and forth too rapidly. The disadvantage of this system is that for any given amount of friction introduced, the amputee is limited to only one cadence.* However, much better control can be obtained by taking advantage of the resistance provided when a fluid is forced through an orifice. Thus there are three main methods of controlling the shank during the swing phase of walking: *Mechanical Lock, Mechanical Friction,* and *Fluid Resistance.*

### *Mechanical Lock*

When a knee joint is locked during the swing phase, the amputee must vault over the prosthesis during the stance phase and swing the rigid leg through during the swing phase, actions that require unnecessary amounts of energy. Although designed to reduce the chance of a fall, when falling does occur, it is apt to be more dangerous than when it occurs as a result of the knee buckling. Thus, a mechanical lock is used very rarely, usually for an infirm patient who wants to stand a bit and move about in a very limited manner. Mechanical locks for this purpose are designed so that the lock engages automatically when the amputee rises to a fully standing position. The lock can be disengaged manually when the amputee desires to return to a seat-

*Theoretically, this problem can be ameliorated by changing the amount of mechanical friction that is applied as the shank swings back and forth, but designs incorporating this feature have failed to win acceptance.

ed position. The control for this can be located in any position that makes it easy for the amputee to manipulate.

### *Mechanical Friction*

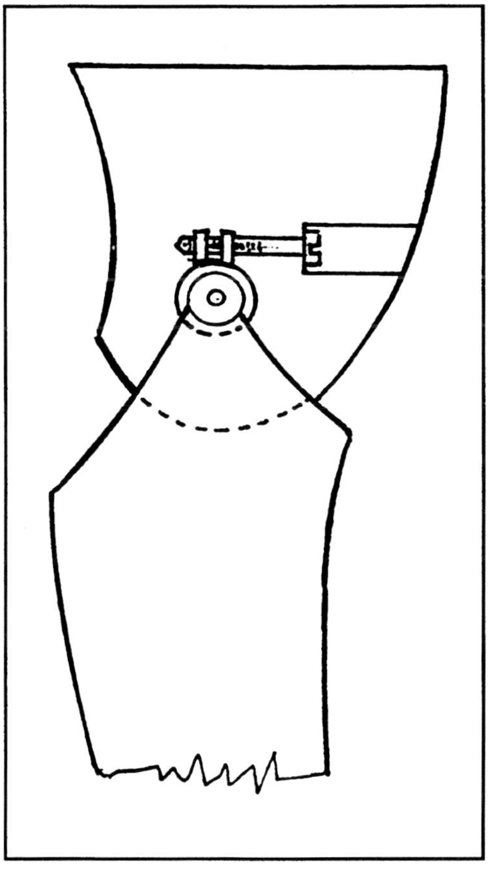

Figure 43. Schematic of a simple constant friction swing-phase control for an artificial knee. The amount of friction is regulated by turning the screw which determines the degree of friction between the bank and knee axle.

The simplest way to provide resistance about a knee joint is to tighten a concentric band about the axle (Figure 43). This method and other comparable systems are called "constant friction" systems.

Although constant friction systems served a large proportion of the transfemoral amputee population for many years, they are prescribed much less frequently now since more effective alternatives are widely available.

### *Fluid Control Units*

Resistance to the flow of fluids through an orifice, either liquid and gaseous, increases with velocity at a rate that compares favorably with the changes in resistance required to control the shank during the swing phase of walking. Therefore, knee units using this principle permit the most normal appearing gait at this time in our technological development. Hydraulic fluid used in aircraft and automobiles is the most common liquid employed, while ambient atmospheric air is quite satisfactory for use in pneumatic units.

#### Hydraulic Swing Phase Control Units

The first commercially successful system for control of the shank during the swing phase of walking was the "Hydra-Cadence" Leg (Figure 44)(58) in which knee and ankle motion are coordinated to

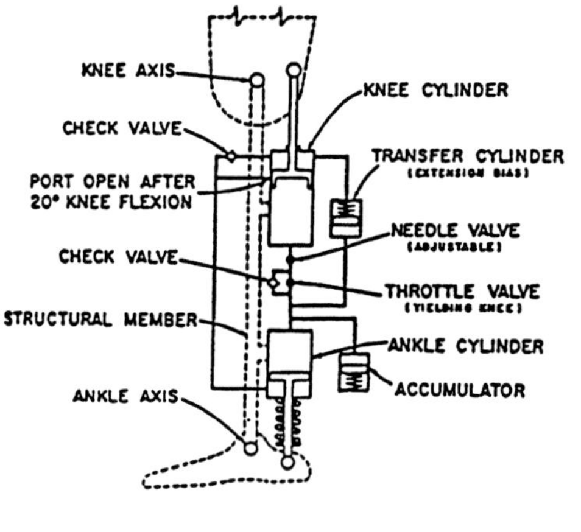


Figure 44. The Hydra-Cadence leg. Left, schematic of the hydraulic system. Courtesy of Artificial Limbs. Right, the hydra-cadence leg with the cosmetic cover removed.

give greater toe clearance during the swing phase. The designer did not have the benefit of the locomotion data that were developed later, but nevertheless the user of the Hydra-Cadence Leg could vary his gait. Although one had to accept the whole system, the cosmesis that could be obtained often left something to be desired, and while considerable maintenance was required, the "Hydra-Cadence" was accepted by the Veterans Administration and many of its beneficiaries as a worthwhile advance in prosthetics. The Hydra-Cadence Leg is still available today (58) for those who have special needs that can be provided by the foot and ankle system and for replacement when a previous wearer feels that he or she does not want to make a change to another design. Otherwise, very few Hydra-Cadence units are prescribed today.

The first successful hydraulic swing-phase control unit where the design was based on scientific data is the Mauch swing phase unit (Figure 45)(38) in which the number of orifices through which the fluid

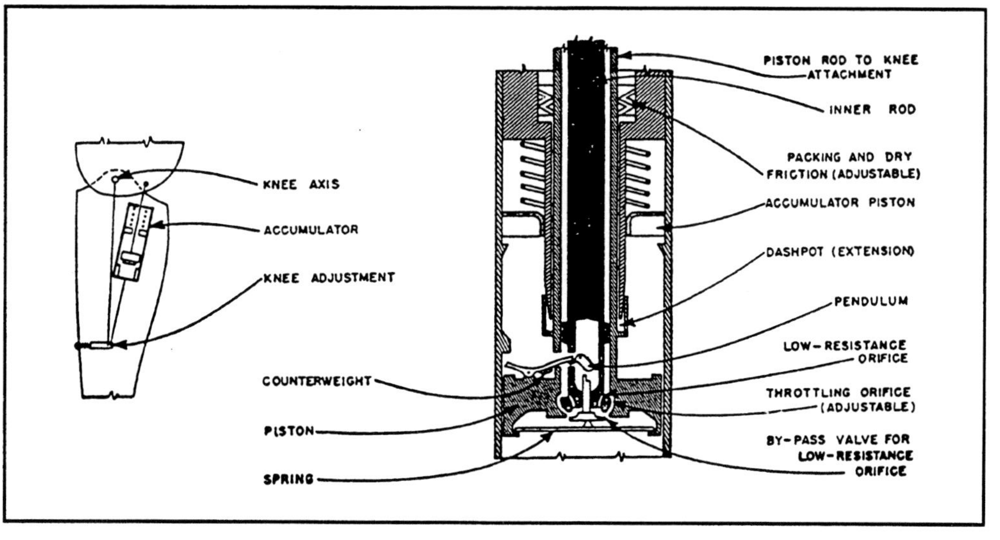


Figure 45. Schematic of Mauch S n 'S Hydraulic Knee Unit that provides automatic control of the artificial leg in both swing and stance phases of walking, and during standing. Courtesy Dept. of Veterans Affairs.

can pass changes as the shank moves through its range of motion. The Mauch units use a cylinder-and-piston system in which the end of the piston rod is attached to the thigh unit posteriorly to the knee, and the cylinder is attached to the shank so that the piston forces oil through an array of orifices as the shank is moved forward. This unit is still available today but it is more commonly used as part of the Mauch S 'n S in which a stance phase control device has been incorporated.

The Mauch swing control system is still one of the most sophisticated units in use but there are also available designs that make compromises between function on the one hand and costs on the other. Many of these units are interchangeable with the Mauch units and therefore with each other. Several manufacturers offer shank units (Figure 46) for endoskeletal prostheses that make it quite possible to interchange a number of systems, a feature that permits a user to select a unit that suits his or her needs best.

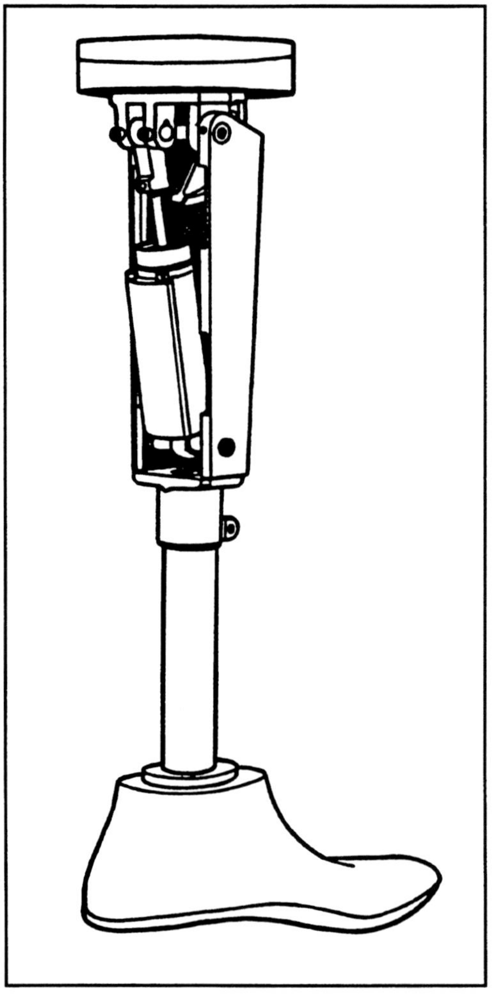

Figure 46. Typical endoskeletal system that allows interchange of different types of knee control units - hydraulic, pneumatic, or constant friction. The frame remains as a part of the prothesis. Courtesy of Dept. of Veterans Affairs.

To reduce weight, designers have also made available very small hydraulic swing phase units that are part of endoskeletal systems, and therefore are not interchangeable.

PNEUMATIC SWING-PHASE CONTROL KNEE UNITS

Designers have also used air, or pneumatics to control the shank during the swing phase. Units used today are commonly of the piston and cylinder type and are interchangeable with most of the other swing phase control units (23). Pneumatic swing-phase units are usually restricted to light-to-moderate duty applications, although recent microprocessor-controlled units are suitable for a greater range of walking speeds.

### *Stance Phase Control*

Methods for controlling the knee joint during standing and the stance phase of walking can be achieved in at least five ways:

- Alignment in the Sagittal Plane
- Mechanical Lock
- Weight-Actuated Brake
- Polycentric Linkage
- Fluid Resistance

#### *ALIGNMENT*

Stability during standing can be achieved by placing the center of the single axis knee joint behind, or posterior to, the weightbearing line (Figure 47). The degree of stability is proportional to the distance the knee center is placed posterior to the weightbearing line. However, the more stable the leg, the more difficult it is for the amputee to flex the knee when moving into the swing phase of walking. Amputees with long stumps and good hip extensor muscles need only a small amount of alignment stability, while those with shorter stumps and less control of the hip extensors will require more. Alignment stability and constant friction swing-phase control units were used together for many years, even for active amputees, until the advent of more sophisticated devices. Some degree of alignment stability is still required even with the more sophisticated stance control devices.

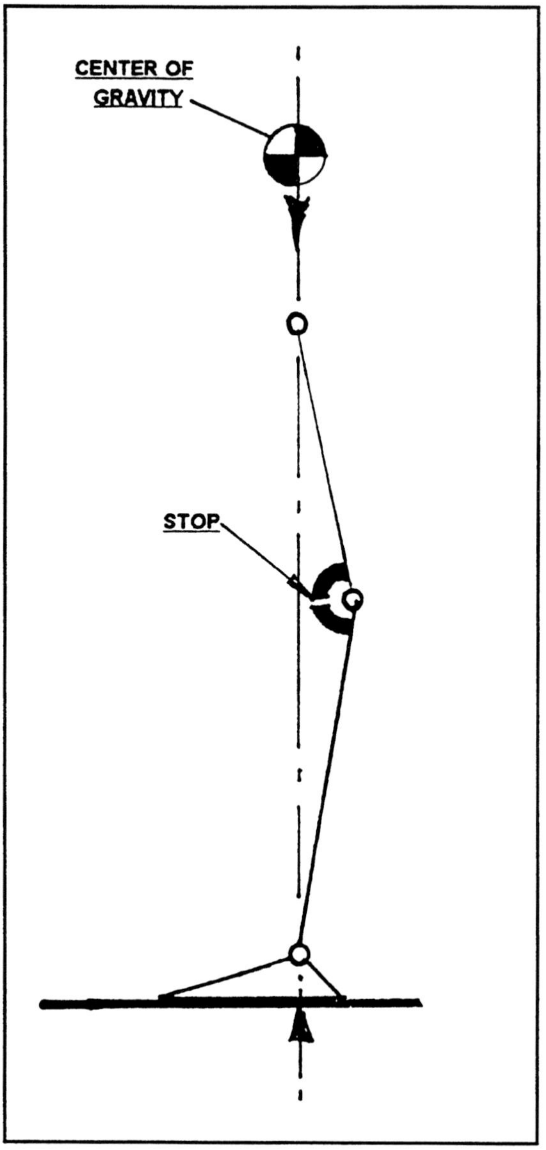


Figure 47. Schematic showing principle of "alignment stability." When the axis of the knee unit is located posterior to the weight line (path of the force from the center of gravity to the floor) and a stop is employed, the joint will not buckle.

### *Mechanical Lock*

For amputees who are weak or who have problems of balance, a mechanical lock can be used to provide stability during standing and the swing phase of walking. The most common design is a lock which engages automatically when the amputee assumes an erect posture and can be unlocked manually by pulling on a lanyard that can be placed in any convenient location on the prosthesis. Of course, with a locked knee, the gait is grossly abnormal, but such an arrangement is a relatively inexpensive way to make it possible for infirm patients to stand and move about a bit rather than being confined to a chair or bed. It must be remembered though that a fall with a locked knee can be even more dangerous than a fall from a buckling knee.

### *Weight-Actuated Brake*

The idea of using a brake actuated brake when the amputee bears his weight on the prosthesis to control the knee during stance phase seems to have come from Germany soon after World War II. The most successful import was originally marketed as the Otto Bock "Safety Knee" in which two bolts in the knee unit are arranged so that weight-bearing causes the upper part of the knee unit to pivot slightly to cause a braking action between thigh and shank (Figure 48, Left). The original units, which are still available today (46) have been renamed "Stance Control" knee units, were installed in wooden knee and shin "set-ups" and incorporated a mechanical friction and extension assist device. The concept of weight-activated braking to supplement alignment stability is also incorporated into several small, streamlined designs especially for use with endoskeletal systems (Figure 48, Right)(5,46).

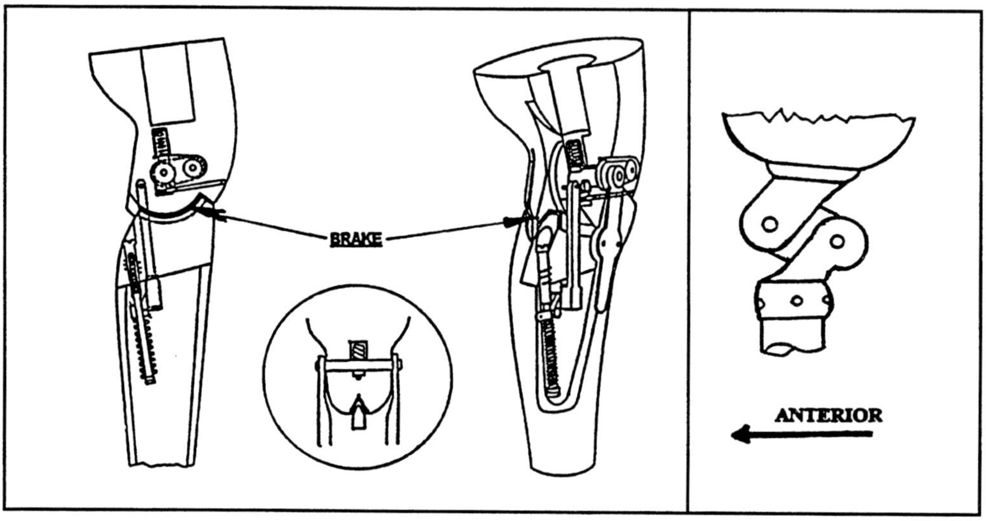


Figure 48. Left, the original "safety knee" manufactured by Otto Bock for use in crustacean type prostheses. When weight is placed on the leg the upper part of the knee pivots downward into a groove to provide a braking action. The control of swing phase is effected by constant friction and a spring for extension bias. Courtesy of *Artificial Limbs.* Right, The same functions embodied in a unit suitable for endoskeletal construction. These units are now designated "Stance Control" knees.

The obvious functional disadvantage of a weight-activated stance-control knee unit is the need to unload completely the leg before flexion can occur. This affects the gait of all users to some degree, and precludes its application in bilateral cases because it makes sitting from a standing position impossible from a practical standpoint.

An additional factor to be considered is the inevitable decrease in braking quality owing to wearof the parts. Finally, falling with a knee which will not bend presents risks similar to using a locked knee.

## *Polycentric Linkage*

By using four or more "bars" linked together so that they can pivot about each other, it is possible to build a device in which the center of rotation of the knee can be made to move through a path that enhances the ability of the amputee to control the knee while standing and during the stance phase of walking by flexion and extension of the hip (Figure 49)(13,49). Another feature inherent in the design is an increase in toe clearance during the swing phase of walking.

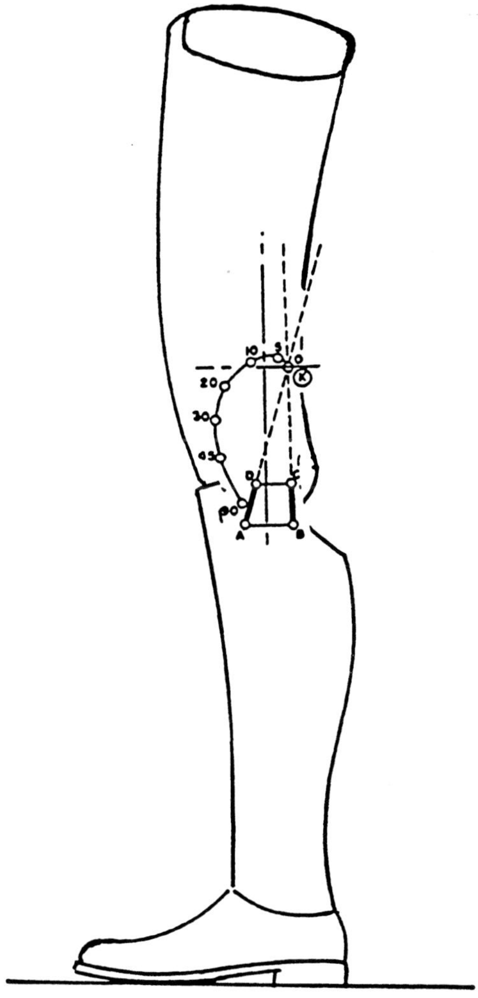

Figure 49. Schematic showing how a four-bar linkage can be designed to provide a path of instant centers of rotation of a knee joint that enhances the control of the leg by use of the stump during standing and the stance phase of walking. The instant center of rotation is found at the intersection of the center lines of the anterior and posterior links. The figures on the curve indicate the amount of knee flexion present for that position of the center of rotation. Small changes in the length and position of the links can result in significant changes in the characteristics of the curve. The curve depicted here is much like the curve found in the human knee. Courtesy of *Artificial Limbs.*

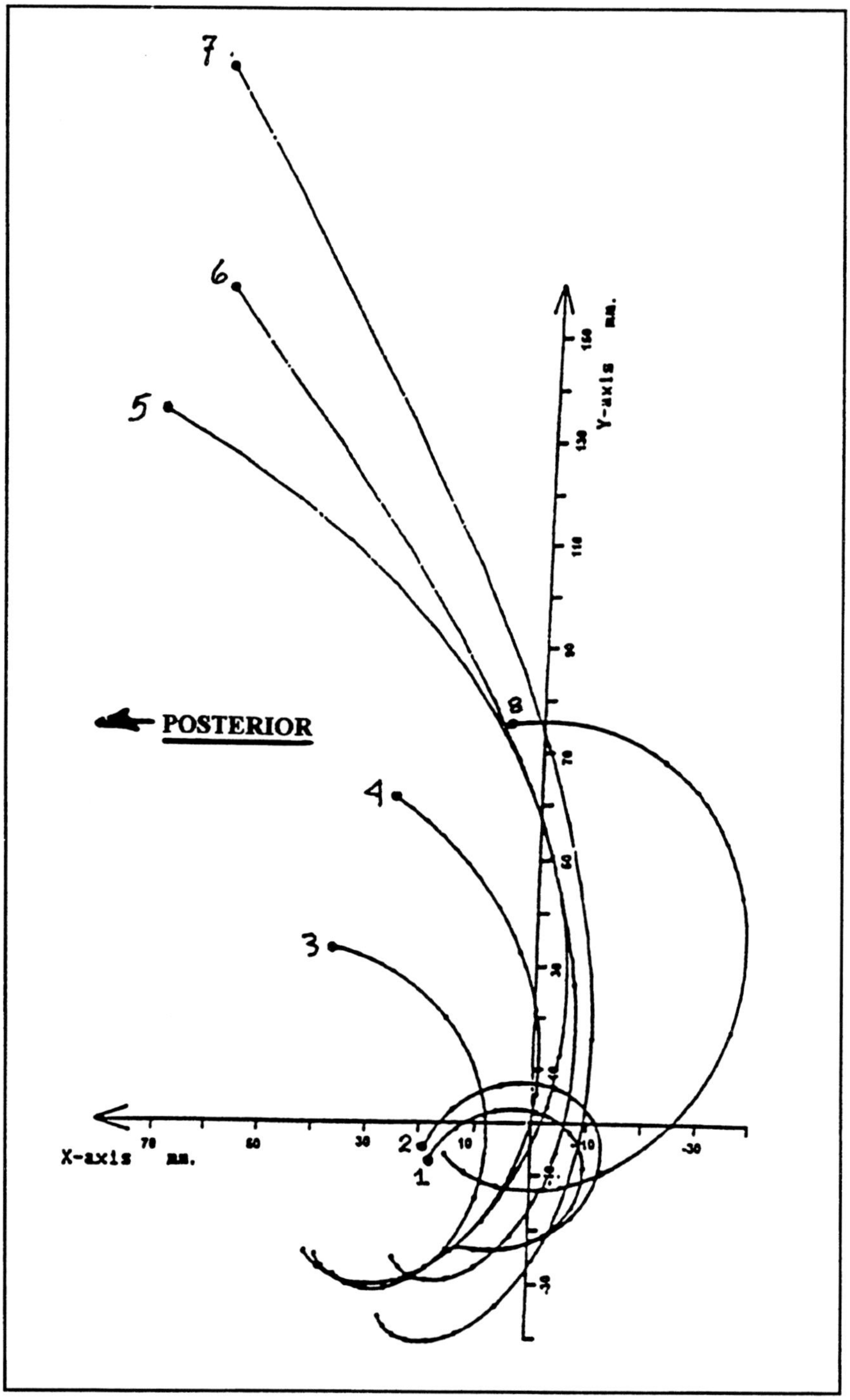


Figure 50. Graph showing the variation of the path of instant centers of rotation for eight different four-bar commercially available polycentric knees. Note that the center of rotation in full extension is posterior to the load line (for alignment stability) and most are located in the thigh region well above the junction of the tibia and femur. Modified from (8) with permission.

In most designs available today, the center of rotation of the knee at full extension is located well above the level of the knee and posterior to the weight, or force, line from which it moves anteriorly and distally as the knee is flexed (Fig. 50). Each design seems to provide a different path of instant centers and the optimal path has yet to be defined. While it is possible to use polycentric knees with exoskeletal construction, present designs are almost universally used with endoskeletal structures. Hydraulic, pneumatic, and mechanical friction swing phase control units can be accommodated by most of the polycentric designs available today, and many have specially designed swing-phase units built in.

At the present time, a polycentric knee unit with hydraulic swing-phase control (Figure 51) in an endoskeletal leg is a very popular prescription for relatively active amputees.

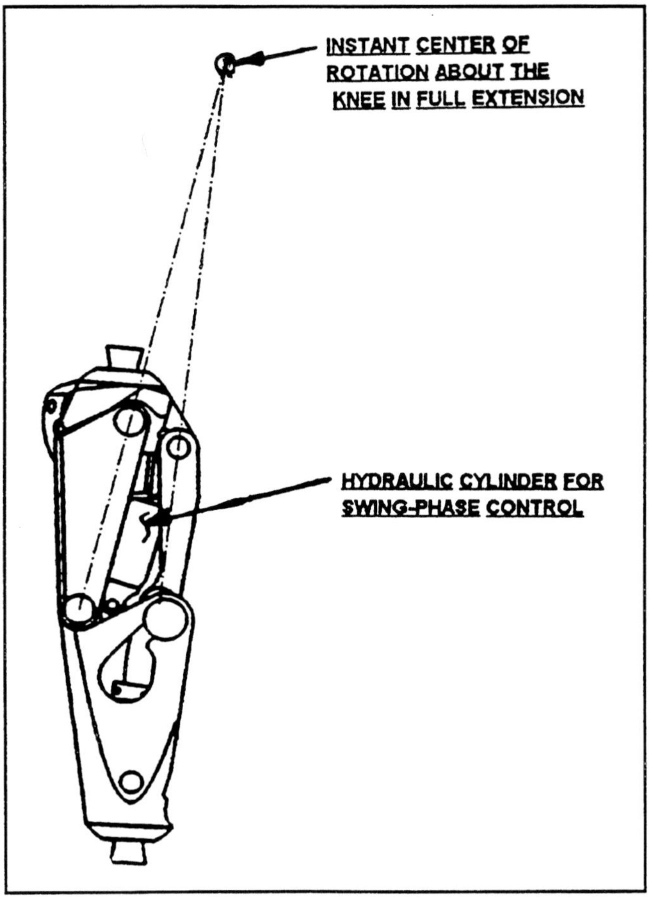


Figure 51. A knee unit with a polycentric four-bar linkage for stance phase control and a hydraulic swing-phase control device. Redrawn from *Otto Bock Orthopadic Industries* with permission.

## *Fluid Resistance*

### *Hydraulic*

The Mauch S'n'S Knee (38) was for many years the only swing-phase control unit that provides stance-phase control as well, a feature that causes a braking action to occur automatically when there is a tendency for the knee to buckle, but recently a similar unit has been made available by another manufacturer (10). In addition to its automatic features, the S 'n S and similar units permit the user to select a "free swing" mode for bicycling or other situations, and a fully locked mode for long periods of standing. Still another swing-and-stance control unit has been introduced recently (46). This new design (Figure 52) employs a rotary type unit that operates about the knee axis instead of a piston and cylinder to achieve the desired characteristics. Although the weight, size, and costs limit somewhat their acceptance, these sophisticated units are well received by active amputees who can take advantage of their complex features.

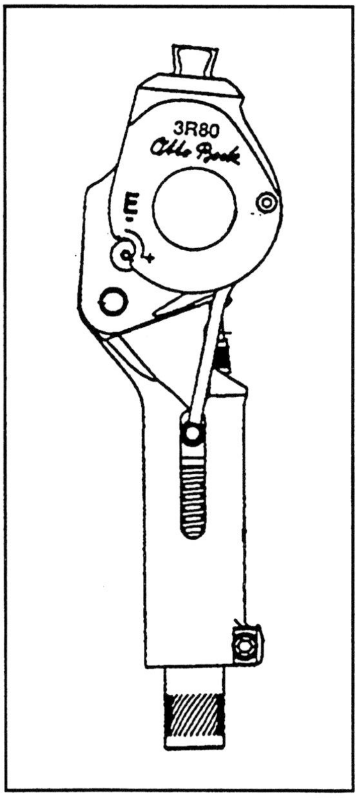


Figure 52. A swing-and-stance-phase control knee unit that uses a rotor about the knee axis instead of a piston and cylinder. Courtesy of *Otto Bock Orthopaedic Industry*.

## PROSTHESES FOR DISARTICULATION AT THE KNEE

Disarticulation at the knee through the years has posed difficult problems for prosthetists trying to provide this type of amputee with a satisfactory device, and lack of a suitable prosthesis discouraged surgeons from using the knee disarticulation procedure even though it has many advantages, including less effects on the patient during the operation and the ability of the resulting stump to bear weight distally. The most troubling problem was finding a method of controlling motion about the knee when there was apparently no space available for the installation of a unit to provide adequate control. Another troubling problem was fabrication of a socket that could be donned easily while accepting the bulbous distal portion of the typical stump.

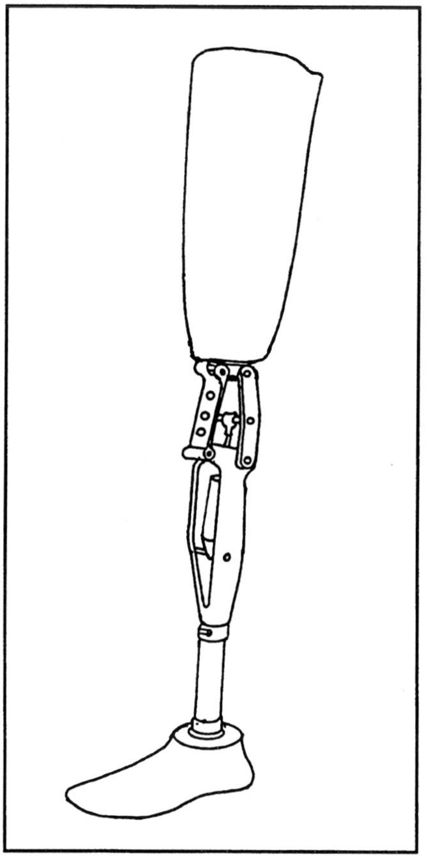

Figure 53. Prosthesis for knee-disarticulation case. The use of a four-bar polycentric knee located distal to the stump permits a fairly normal swing phase while providing excellent control of the prosthesis during standing and the stance phase of walking. Various swing-phase control units can be used with the polycentric units. Shown here is a hydraulic swing-phase control unit.

The first of these problems was solved by use of a four-bar polycentric joint that could be installed below the distal end of the socket, that is, within the shank area of the prosthesis, and still provide a location of the center of rotation above the level of the condyles (Figure 53). In fact, the OHC unit (34), the first of its kind, provided a center of rotation well above the condyles, thus making control of the knee joint considerably easier during stance phase while increasing toe clearance during the swing phase. Today, except for a few instance where excessively hard use is expected, polycentric knee units are universally prescribed for amputees with a knee disarticulation.

Plastic sockets with "windows" or with elastic foam in the space just above the condyles, as used in prostheses for Syme's amputation, have replaced the molded leather sockets of yesterday that used laced openings to accommodate the bulbous stumps.

## PROSTHESES FOR HIP DISARTICULATION AND TRANSPELVIC AMPUTEES

The hip-disarticulation amputee is almost always provided with a plastic socket either laminated or heat formed over a modified plaster model of the "stump" or lower torso mounted on endoskeletal thigh and shank sections. The Canadian system (Figure 54), where the "hip" joint is mounted transversely on the anterior aspect of the socket, is universally employed. Several mechanical systems are available to replace the elastic straps used in the original designs. Because most amputees who have lost all or nearly all of a lower limb are not very active, a single-axis knee unit with a constant friction swing-phase control and a SAFE foot usually meets their requirements, but it is not rare for a hip disarticulee to make good use of more sophisticated knees and feet. For those patients who feel the need for more security than that afforded by the conventional system, a hip joint with a manual lock is available.

When the endoskeletal hardware is covered with foam rubber and an elastic stocking the cosmetic effect is quite natural.

Prescription for transpelvic amputees is the same as that for the hip disarticulee, but the suspension of the socket requires some modification from that of the hip case (Figure 55).

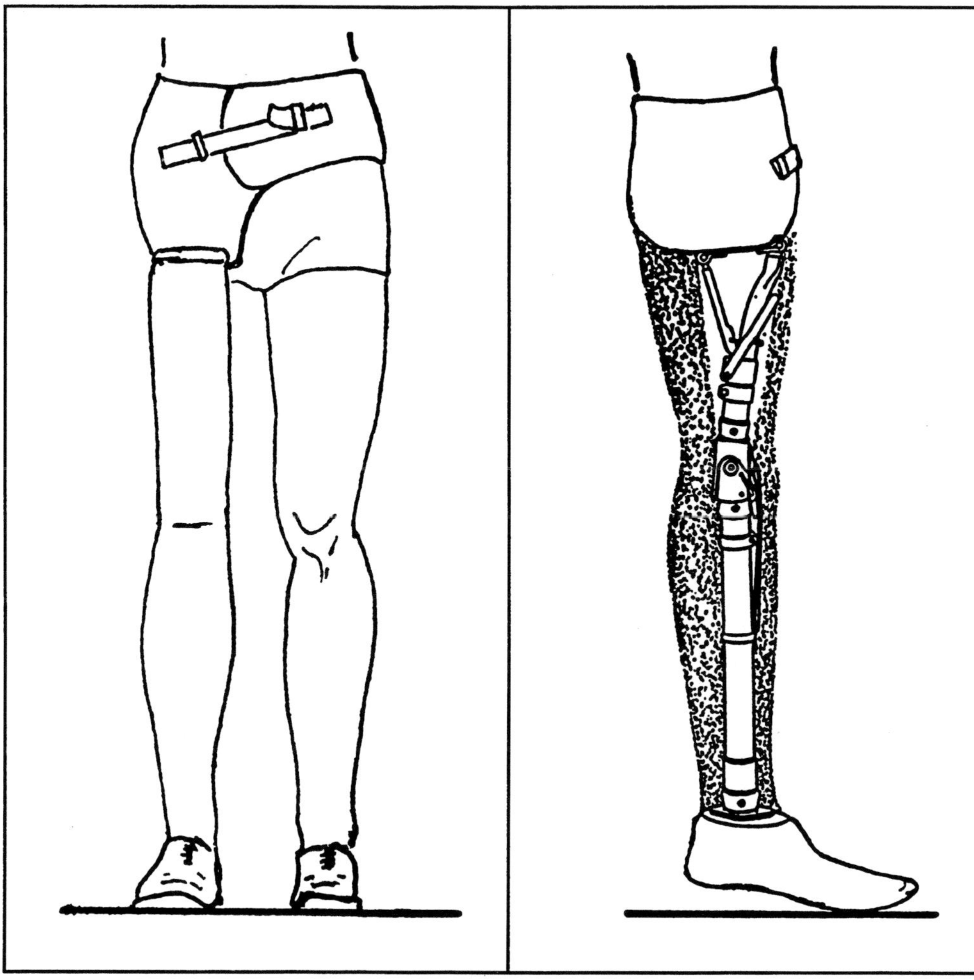

Figure 54. Typical Prosthesis for the hip disarticulation case. Most knee units can be used, but emphasis is usually on using the lighter units.

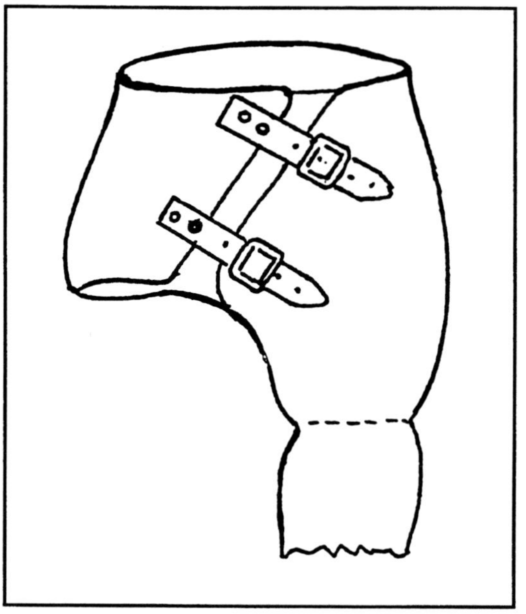

Figure 55. Typical socket for transpelvic prostheses. Note the angle of the opening of the socket required to achieve a balance of forces between the prosthesis and the patient.

## SPECIAL CONSIDERATIONS FOR BILATERAL LOWER LIMB AMPUTEES

Obviously, standing and walking with two artificial legs requires much more than double the skill and energy, and thus training, than when only one leg is affected. The principal problem is stability. The higher the levels of amputation, the more the problem. Bilateral lower limb amputees often develop hip flexion and abduction contractures aggravated by prolonged sitting and bedrest. Contractures should be avoided because they often prevent achieving alignment stability, making manual knee locks necessary and causing an awkward, inefficient gait. Fitting artificial limbs as early as possible should be emphasized, not only to reduce the tendency of contractures to occur, but also to keep the amputee active and easier to keep in condition to use artificial limbs. The use of two knees with weightbearing brakes such as the "Safety Knee" is contraindicated because going from a standing position to sitting safely with two of these devices is impossible.

To assess the potential ability of the bilateral transfemoral amputee, to aid in prevention of contractures, and to promote a healthy stump, and thus accelerate rehabilitation, it is desirable to begin with "stubbies," a set of sockets fitted with bottom pieces that interfere as little as possible with locomotion, yet provide a distal surface that aids in stability while standing (Figure 56).

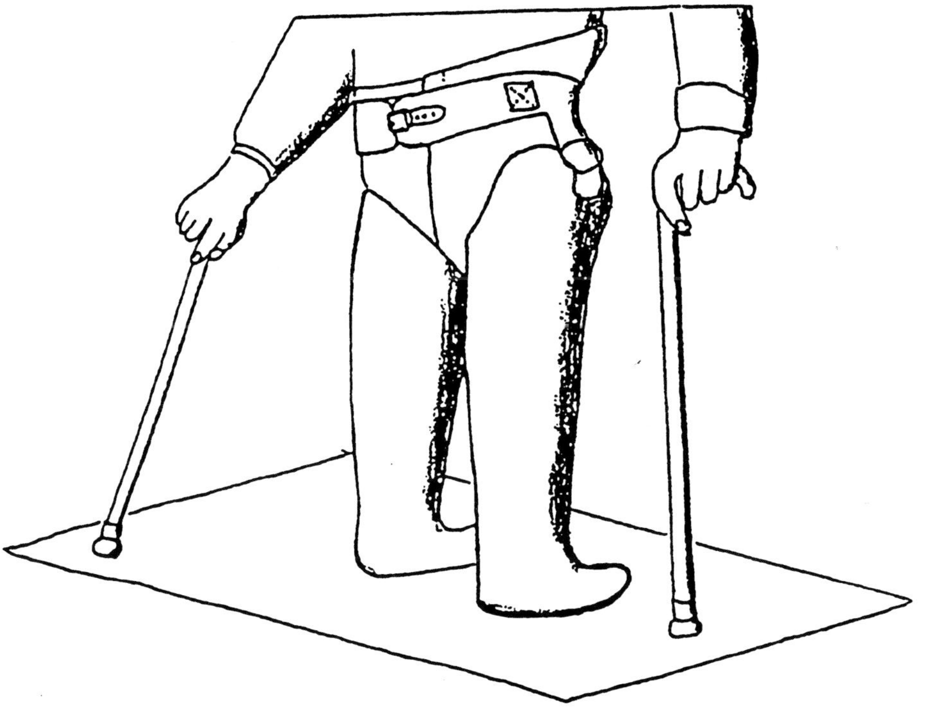

Figure 56. "Stubbies" for bilateral transfemoral amputee. There is as yet no standardized shape for the "feet." Each set it designed to meet the balance and locomotion problems for the individual patient.

Except for those knees that brake or lock upon weightbearing, practically all the knee joints available can be used with bilateral cases. Weight is even more important than with cases with only one amputation, and thus, prostheses should be as light as practicable. The length of prostheses for bilateral cases can be varied to suit the circumstances. When stability appears to be a serious problem, the center of gravity of the amputee can be lowered by reducing the length of the legs for the initial phase of training and lengthened later, if desired, so that the patient can attain the height present before the amputations.

Although it is not unusual for an amputee with two intact knee joints to walk without canes, nearly all bilateral amputees who have lost either one or both knees require at least one cane.

## PRESCRIPTION NOTES

To provide guidelines for prescribers, the Medicare Program in the U.S. has adopted a functional classification system (54) as follows:

**Level 0:** Patient does not have the ability or potential to ambulate or transfer safely with or without assistance and a prosthesis does not enhance their quality of life or mobility.

**Level 1:** Patient has the ability or potential to use a prosthesis for transfers or ambulation on level surfaces at fixed cadence. Typical of the limited and unlimited household ambulator.

**Level 2:** Patient has the ability or potential for ambulation with the ability to traverse low level environmental barriers such as curbs, stairs, or uneven surfaces. Typical of the limited community ambulator.

**Level 3:** Patient has the ability or potential for ambulation with variable cadence. Typical of the unlimited community ambulator who has the ability to traverse most environmental barriers and may have vocational, therapeutic, or exercise activity that demands prosthetic utilization beyond simple locomotion.

**Level 4:** Patient has the ability or potential for prosthetic ambulation that exceeds basic ambulation skills, exhibiting high impact, stress, or energy levels. Typical of the prosthetic demands of the child, active adult, or athlete.

Under Medicare rules Level 0 patients are not provided with a prosthesis, but clinicians must be careful when applying this rule, since the act of being fitted sometimes provides the patient with the will to improve his or her lot, and the activity level increases progressively.

Level 1 patients are restricted to use of a SACH foot or a single-axis foot, and most knee units except for hydraulic and pneumatic units.

Level 2 patients may be provided with a flexible keel foot such as the SAFE foot, but are restricted from receiving hydraulic or pneumatic knee units.

Level 3 patients may be provided with either a multiaxis foot such as the Greissinger, or one of the so-called dynamic response feet such as Carbon Copy II, or the Flex Foot. Level 3 patients can also make use of knee units that are controlled by hydraulic or pneumatic systems.

Level 4 patients may be provided with a prosthesis that best meets his or her vocational and daily living needs.

# UPPER-LIMB PROSTHESIS

A classification of upper-limb amputations is shown in Figure 57.

It seems self-evident that the problems of the upper-limb amputee are quite different from those of persons with lower-limb amputations. With the tremendous potential of the human hand for function, largely untapped in the average person, one unaffected arm and hand can compensate to a large degree for the loss of the function of the other when called upon, and thus the unilateral upper-limb amputee usually does not require a prosthesis to be able to resume a fairly normal

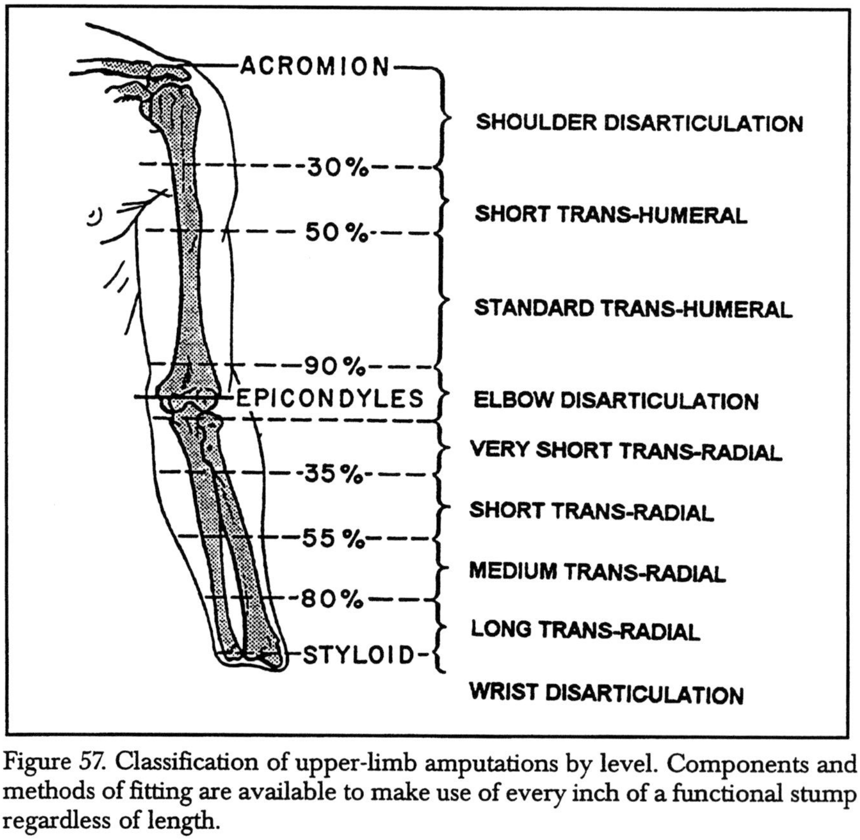


Figure 57. Classification of upper-limb amputations by level. Components and methods of fitting are available to make use of every inch of a functional stump regardless of length.

existence after a relatively brief acclimatizing period, but an artificial leg is required if the lower-limb amputee is to lead a fairly normal life. While there is available a wide variety of components for the prescription of artificial limbs for upper limb amputees, it is not easy to satisfy the needs of individual unilateral amputees, and unfortunately, many patients with a remaining normal arm eventually discard their prostheses. However, individuals who are accustomed to using both arms in relatively strenuous activities such as farm and construction work find an artificial arm indispensable, and, as one might suspect, nearly all bilateral upper-limb amputees appreciate the functions provided by prostheses and generally make full use of their prostheses. Those patients with deficiencies at birth who would seem to need artificial limbs are exceptions.

Perhaps because the proportion of upper-limb amputees to lower-limb amputees is so small, approximately 1:10, and the problems are so difficult, relatively little emphasis has been given during the past several decades to improving upper-limb prostheses, most of the effort in this area being applied to externally-powered devices.

The procedure for providing an artificial arm is very similar to that used for lower-limb prostheses. The prosthetist, working from a prescription, forms a socket over a plaster model of the stump and assembles the arm from components available from manufacturers. The prosthetist then fits the prosthesis to the patient adjusting it so control can be effected in the most efficient manner. Training in efficient use of upper-limb prostheses is extremely important, and is usually carried out by an occupational therapist.

The primary function of the human arm is placement of the hand in a position where it can function (Figure 58). Of the multitude of functions that can be provided by the human hand, studies have shown that palmar prehension is the function used most frequently under ordinary circumstances (55), and, except where cosmesis or appearance is the only reason for using a prosthesis, the design of upper-limb prostheses is based on this fact.

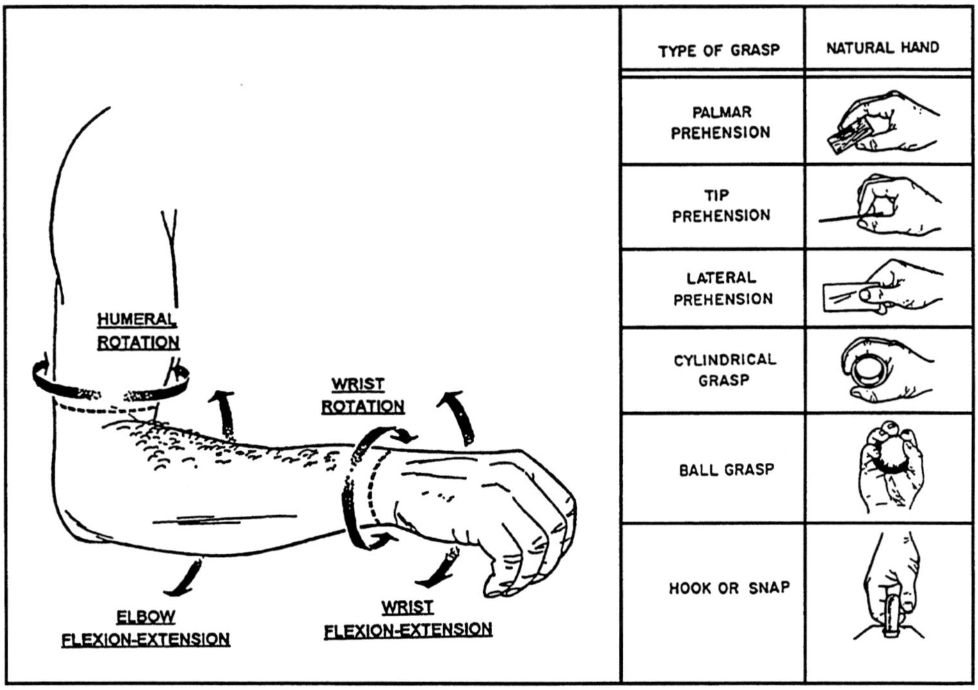


Figure 58. Left, basic functions of the arm and forearm that allow the positioning of the hand for it to function. Not shown is flexion and extension. Right, basic function of the human hand (55). Courtesy of *Artifical Limbs.*

Upper-limb prostheses can be classified as either active or passive. Passive artificial arms have no moving parts except for elbow and shoulder joints that are controlled by the contralateral arm when either or both artificial joints are present. Passive arms are most generally used only for the sake of appearance. However, passive arms can be provided with special devices to perform specific functions such as holding a tool or a ski pole.

Active artificial arms may be actuated and controlled by forces generated entirely by the user or by a source external to the user. Thus, artificial arms are either *body-powered* or *externally-powered.*

Most of the artificial arms fitted at the present time are "body-powered," that is, power is generated by relative motion between two parts of the body, such as flexion about the shoulder joint (Figure 59), which is transmitted from a harness about some portion of the torso through a cable to the component to be actuated or controlled (Figure 60). Although function is limited in body-powered systems, the amount of sensory feedback provided has yet to be achieved in externally-powered systems. In other words, under most circumstances the amputee with the harness system has finer control over the grasping function.

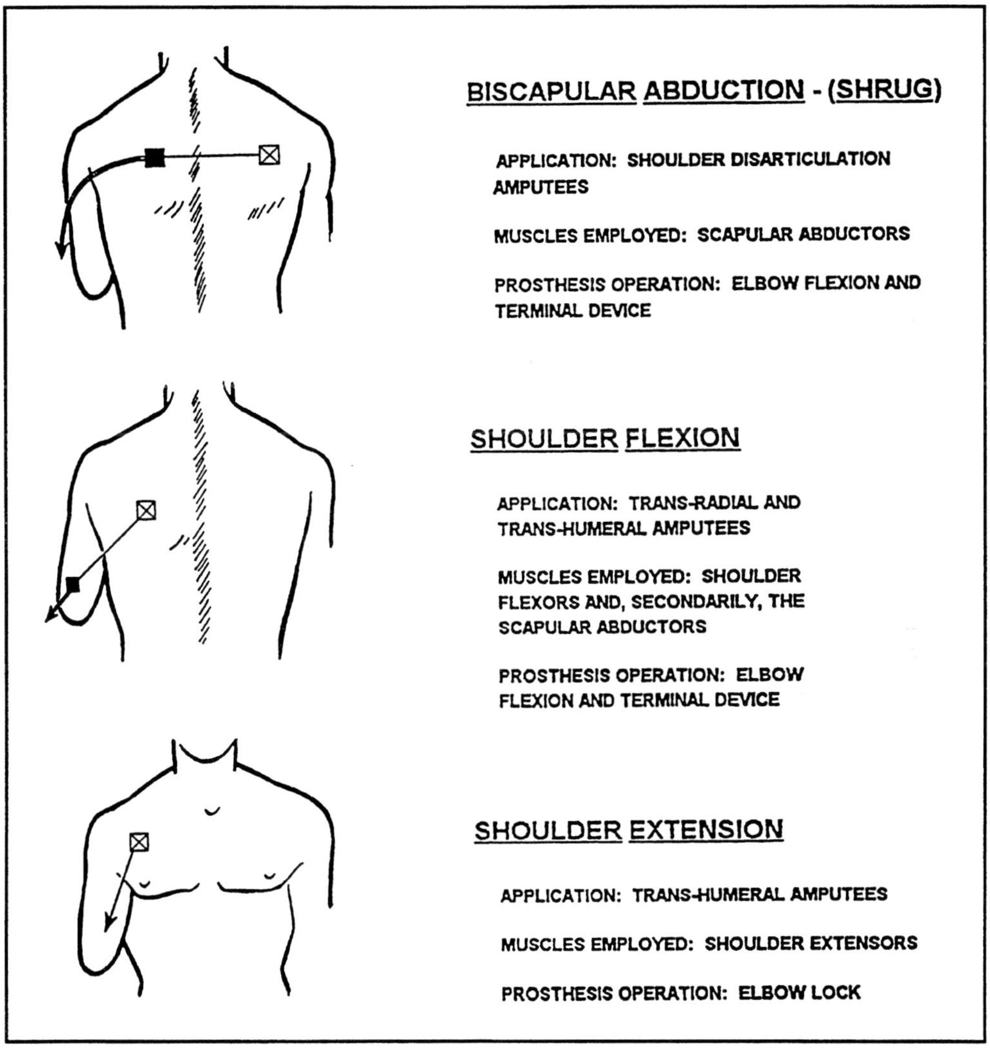


Figure 59. Major harness controls. The points stabilized by harness are beginning points (☒) for the control cable, which passes into a Bowden-type housing at movable points (■). The relative motion is transmitted via the cable (—►) to distal points on the prosthesis. Courtesy of *Artificial Limbs*

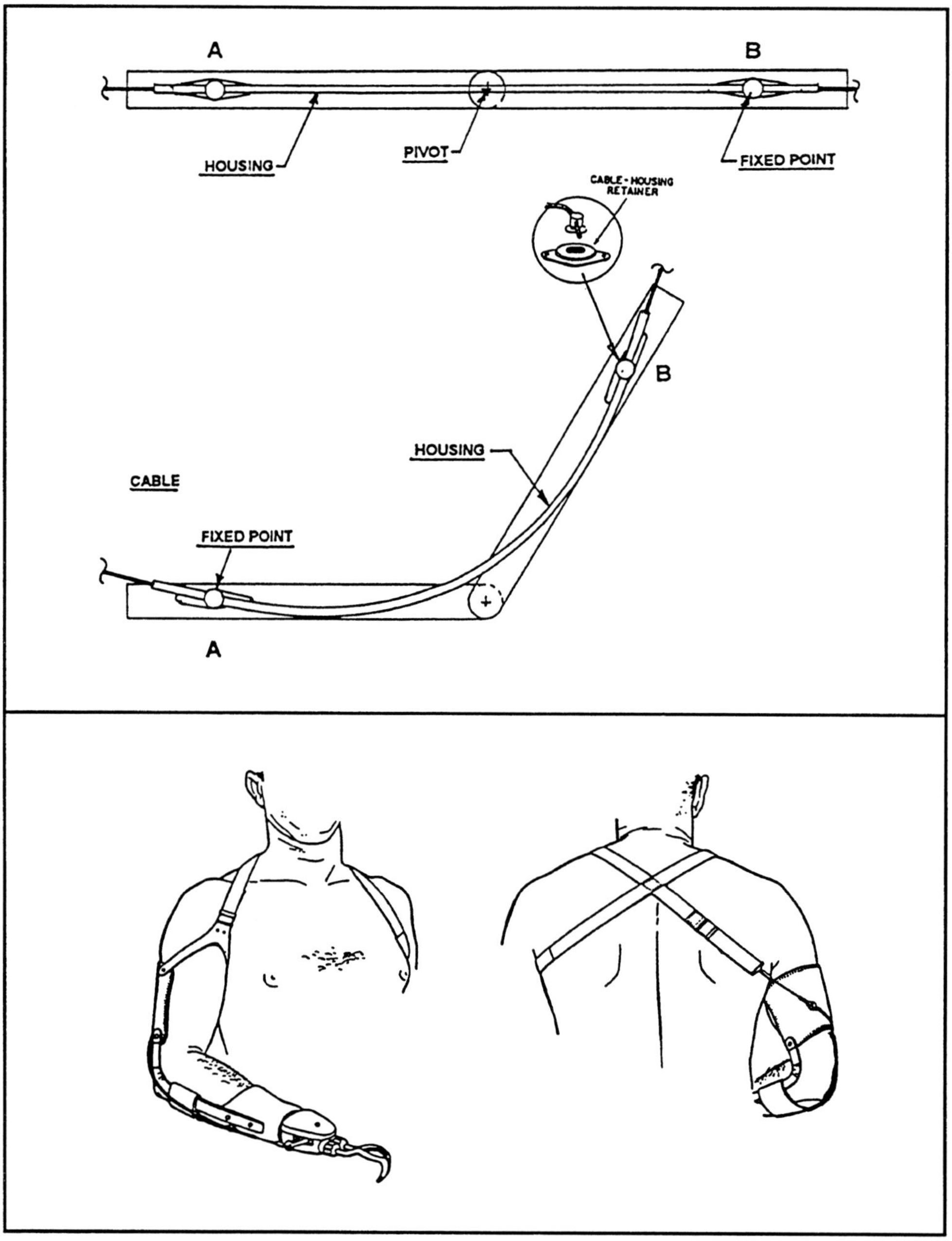


Figure 60. Top, sketch showing the principle of the Bowden cable. When the housing is fixed at two points but rotation of the housing is permitted, the effective length of the cable remains unchanged as one pivots about the other. Thus the dimension AB in the uppermost figure also represents the length AB in the flexed position just below. Bottom, application of the Bowden cable in a harness for actuation and control of a prosthesis for a transradial amputee.

All externally-powered upper-limb prostheses available at the present time use battery-powered electric motors. Components of electric artificial arms may be controlled by either myoelectric signals or by switches activated by subtle body motions.

Just as is the case in lower-limb prosthetics, construction may be either *endoskeletal* or *exoskeletal*, the latter usually reserved for use with passive, or cosmetic, prostheses. Use of the exoskeletal type is almost mandatory for externally-powered systems for storage of batteries and actuators.

A wide array of components is available for fabrication of an upper limb prosthesis to meet many of the needs of individual arm amputees. Compromises must be made, but components to provide substitutes for the hand, wrist, elbow, and to some extent the shoulder joint are in ready supply. In fact, there are available devices that can be used to take advantage of every inch of the upper limb that the surgeon feels is medically feasible to save during amputation.

## BODY-POWERED PROSTHESES

### Components Available

#### *Terminal Devices*

"Terminal devices," or substitutes for the hand, are common to all upper-limb prostheses. There are two broad categories of terminal devices: *hands* and *hooks* (Figure 61). In addition, there are available devices that are intended to provide a specific function such as using a bowling ball or holding a ski pole. Terminal devices are attached to the prosthesis by a "wrist" unit which can be had with a "quick change" mechanism which allows an easy interchange of devices. Many upper-limb amputees use a hook for daily activities but change to a hand for social occasions. An equally important function of wrist units, except for wrist disarticulation and long transradial amputees, is to make it possible for the user to preposition, usually by the contralateral limb, the terminal device in the pronation-supination plane for most effective use.

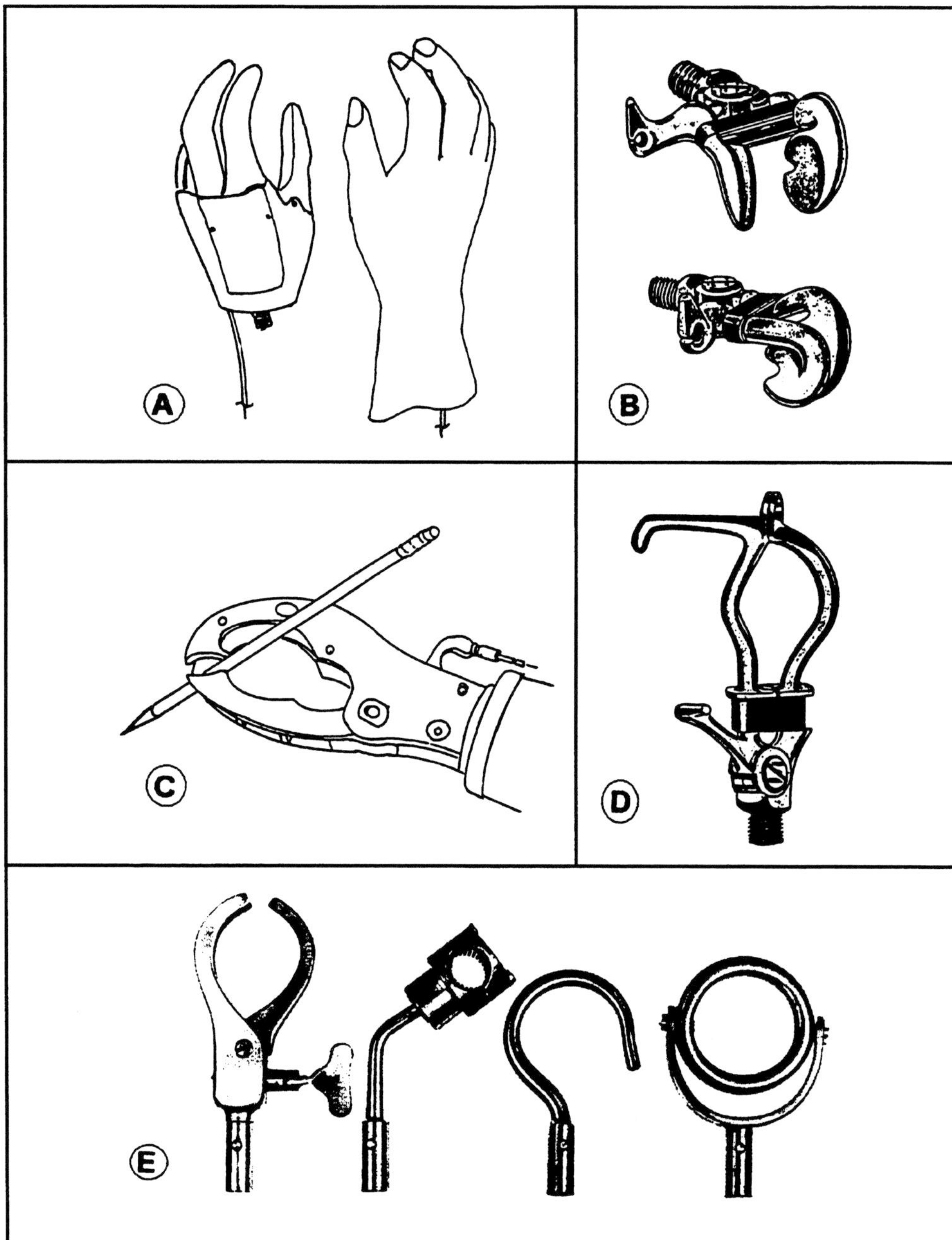


Figure 61. Some of the terminal devices available for upper limb prostheses. (A) Cable controlled artificial hand covered with a realistic plastic glove. (B) Child's voluntary opening "hook", or "wafer", covered with a plastisol to prevent damage (From *Artificial Limbs*). (C) Voluntary closing terminal device from TRS (Courtesy of TRS). (D) Dorrance voluntary opening hook No. 6, a very popular model with carpenters, farmers, and others engaged in strenous two-handed activities. (Courtesy of Hosmer Dorrance Corp.) (E) Examples of single purpose terminal devices. Courtesy of Otto Bock Orthopedic Industry.

Terminal devices may be either active or passive. Passive artificial hands are used almost entirely for appearance, although some models permit a limited ability to hold or to carry objects. The most realistic passive, or cosmetic, hands are custom made for a specific patient, but an acceptable alternative may be had from an array of "off-the-shelf" models. A soft foam hand selected from a wide range of sizes for either male or female configurations can be covered with plastic gloves selected from a wide range of tints. For more strenuous users, there is available a "hard" cosmetic hand that does not require a glove. One model is a lightweight shell made of polyvinyl chloride (PVC).

The functions provided by active terminal devices are, naturally, quite limited. In fact, the only active function available is some type of prehension. Schlesinger (53) identified six basic types of hand prehension patterns (Figure 62), and studies conducted at UCLA (55) showed that palmar prehension is the type most used in daily activities (Figure 63). The most popular artificial hands are designed to provide palmar prehension, usually by a force between a stationary thumb and hinged index and middle fingers.

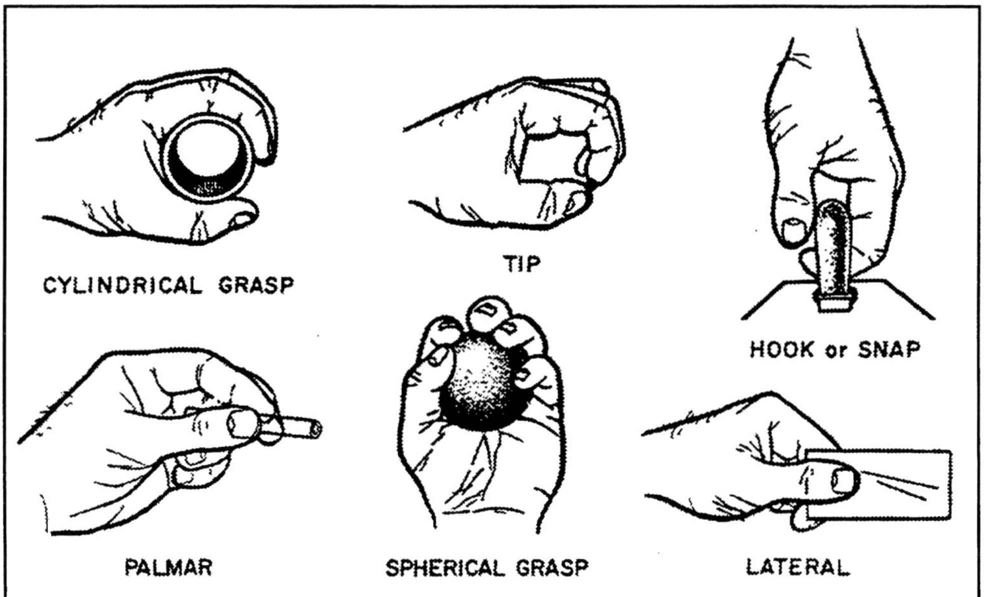


Figure 62. Six major prehension patterns identified by Schlesinger (53).

| FREQUENCY OF PREHENSION PATTERNS | | | |
|---|---|---|---|
| **SERIES** | **OCCURRENCE OF PREHENSION TYPE** | | |
| | **PALMAR (%)** | **TIP (%)** | **LATERAL (%)** |
| **Pick Up** | **50** | **17** | **33** |
| **Hold for Use** | **88** | **2** | **10** |

Figure 63. Frequency of prehension patterns of the human hand in performance of daily activities (55). Courtesy of *Artificial Limbs.*

The limited amount of control that can be had from relative motion between body segments imposes severe restrictions on designers of active terminal devices. Tension transmitted to the terminal device through a cable is the most efficient means of powering an artificial limb component. Such a system requires the use of a spring or other elastic system in the terminal device to return the mechanism to its "resting" position. The limited amount of excursion available can be

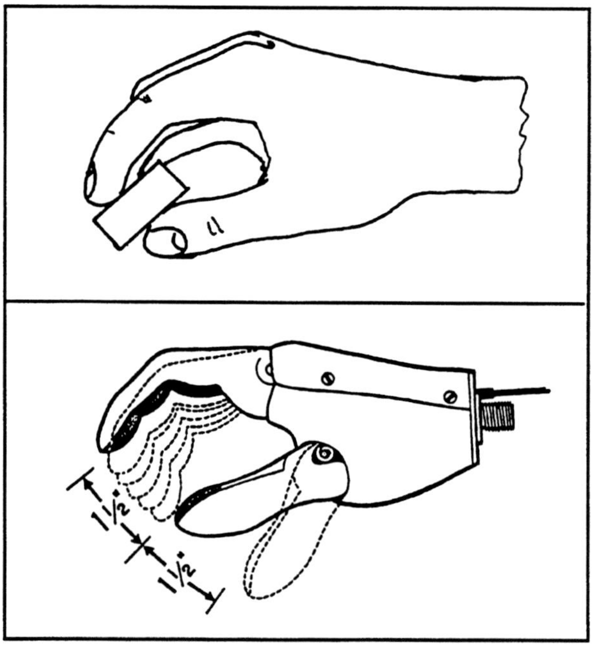

Figure 64. Sketch showing palmar prehension pattern used by many artificial hands. To make maximum use of the excursion availalbe from relative motion between parts of the body, a two position thumb is used. The two position thumb can be set manually from either position to the other by application of pressure on the dorsal side. Lower sketch, courtesy of *Artificial Limbs.*

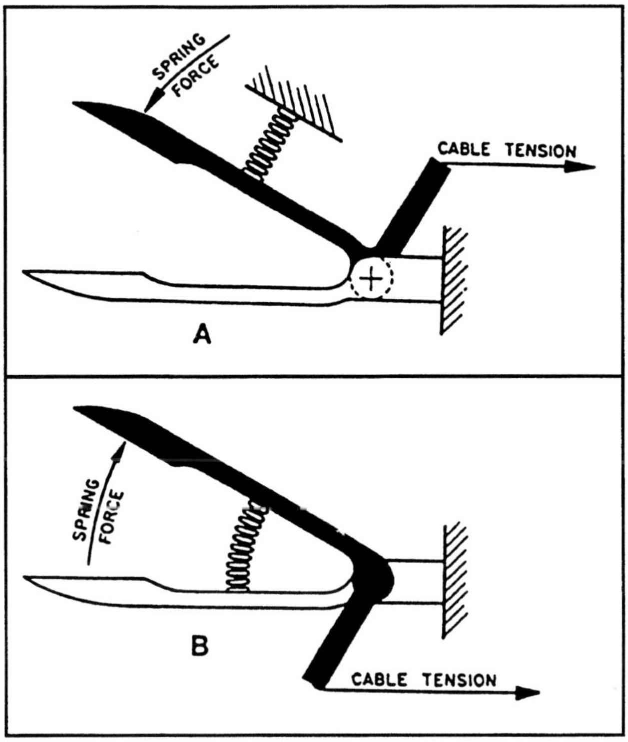


Figure 65. Schematics showing principles of "voluntary opening" (A) and "voluntary closing" (B) terminal device operation. From *Artificial Limbs.*

made more useful by application of the two-position thumb (Figure 64). At the present time, mechanisms for terminal devices are either of the *voluntary-opening* or *voluntary-closing* type (Figure 65). In hands with the voluntary-opening feature, the fingers are opened against a force provided by one or more springs; in most voluntary-opening hooks, one of the fingers is fixed and the other is opened against one or more elastic bands, although springs are used in some designs. A distinct advantage of elastic bands is that the force that best meets the needs of individuals can be achieved easily by selecting the number of elastic bands used.

In voluntary-closing hands, the fingers are usually moved into palmar prehension against a light spring which returns the fingers to the open position ready for the next motion. The fingers are locked in place at a selected force when tension in the control cable is relaxed. The same system has been applied to hooks, but the popular TRS (50,57) model (Figure 61) does not contain this locking feature.

Theoretically, the voluntary-closing terminal devices should be the most useful, but this has not been borne out in practice, no doubt because of some problems inherent in present designs that prevent the voluntary concept from reaching its potential.

Voluntary opening hands are simpler than voluntary closing models and are more popular in spite of their inferior grasping ability. The anthropomorphic models and tinted plastic gloves that appear quite natural are possibly the most appealing attribute of present-day, body-powered hands and the less complicated and less expensive units win out..

The family of voluntary-opening split hooks (Figure 66), the first of which were introduced by Mr. Dorrance about 1909 (15) and refined over the years, still constitutes the most popular terminal devices in use today.

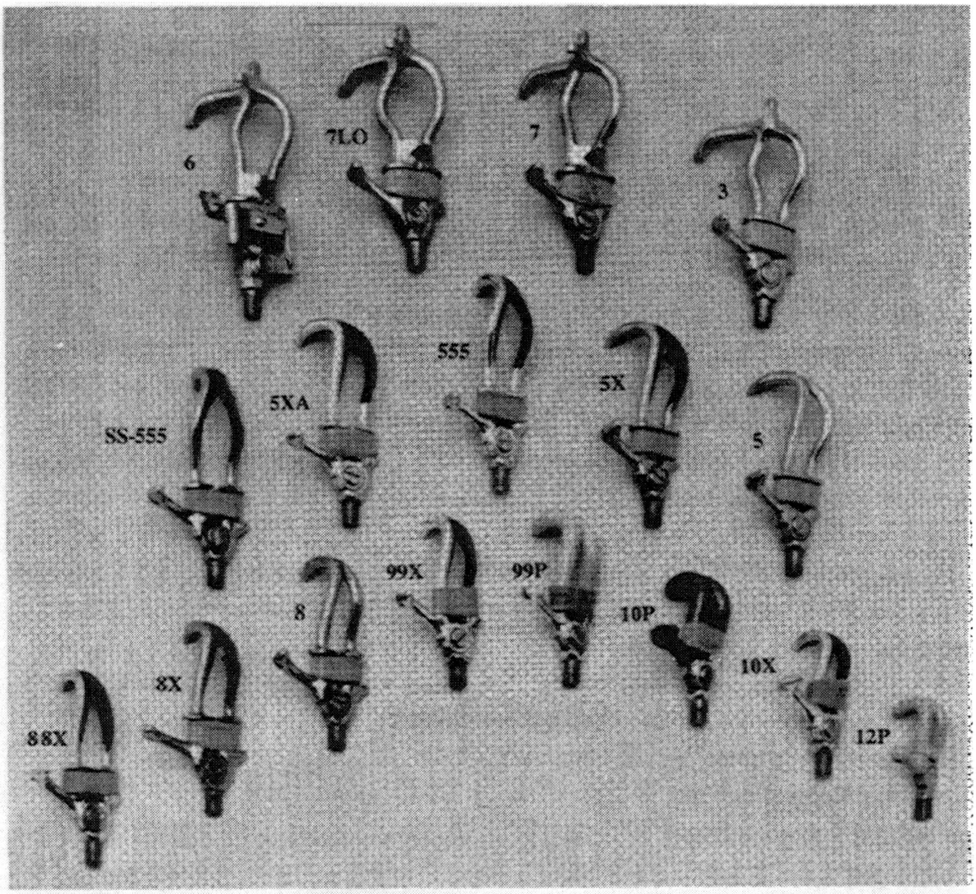


Figure 66. The Family of Dorrance Hooks. Courtesy of Hosmer-Dorrance Corp.

## Wrist Units

Nearly all wrist units provide for attachment of the terminal device to the prosthesis and permit the user to preposition the terminal device in pronation or supination. Several designs allow manually-controlled wrist flexion as well.

The simplest type of wrist unit employs female threads that accept the threaded stud of the terminal device (Figure 67). The orientation of the terminal device about the axis of the wrist unit (pronation-supination) can be controlled manually by the contralateral arm. Friction between nylon or Delrin threads in the wrist unit and the metal threads on the terminal device can be adjusted to the degree required to hold the terminal device in any desired position during operation of the hook or hand (Figure 67). Wrist units featuring the quick change feature allow the terminal device to be locked in the desired position (Figure 67). These designs are, of course, heavier and more expensive than the simple type.

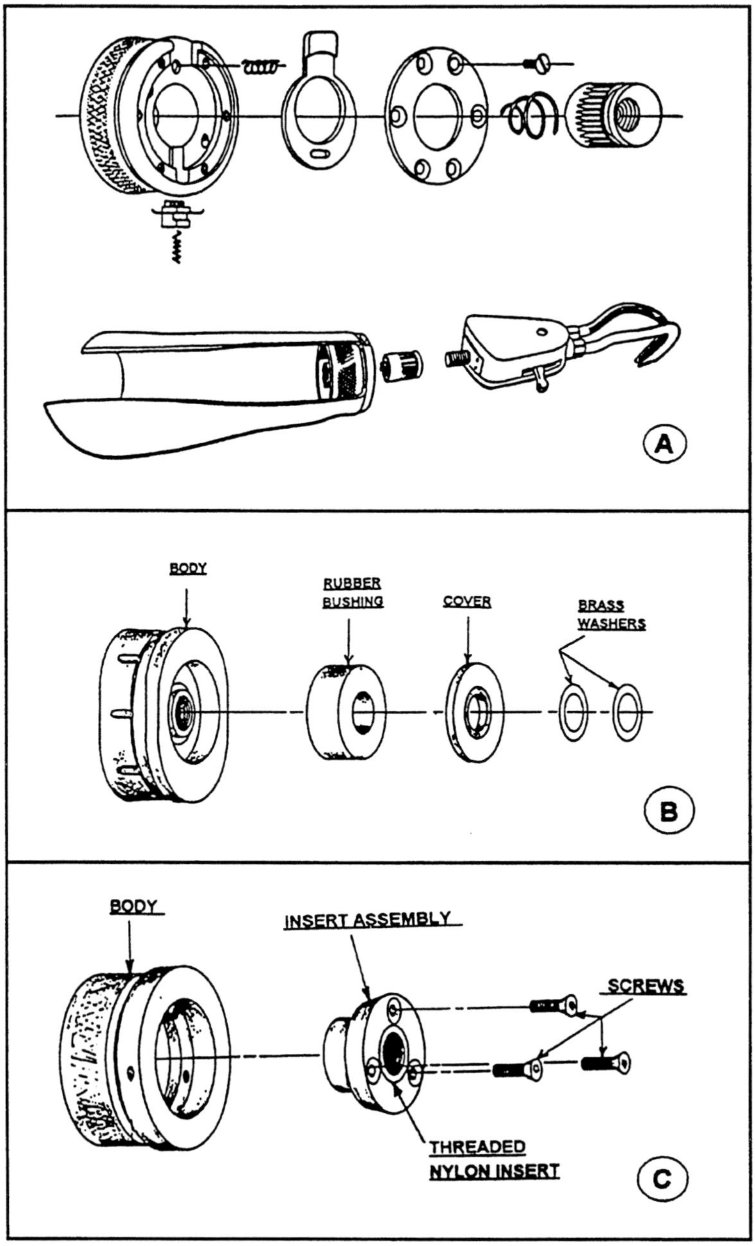


Figure 67. Explosed views of three types of wrist units: (A) Wrist unit for quick interchange of terminal devices. Pronation-supination positioning is maintained by a detent type lock. From Artificial Limbs. (B) Friction-type wrist. Pronation-supination position is maintained by friction between the "cover," rubber bushing and the body of the unit. (C) Friction-type wrist unit in which friction is provided by a threaded nylon insert. The amount of friction can be adjusted with a set screw in the body of the unit. Figs. B&C modified from Hosmer Dorrance (23) with permission.

For the wrist-disarticulation amputee where space is very limited simple, abbreviated, or shortened, units are available.

Devices that permit a certain amount of flexion about the wrist are also available. One design is a separate unit that is introduced between the wrist unit and the terminal device (Figure 68). In another design, the flexion feature is incorporated in the wrist unit itself. Either of three positions can be selected in both designs. For children, a wrist unit with a built-in flexion fixed at 20 degrees is available. Wrist flexion is especially useful in performing many activities of daily living and in certain work situations. A wrist flexion unit should be considered when prescribing for every bilateral upper-limb case.

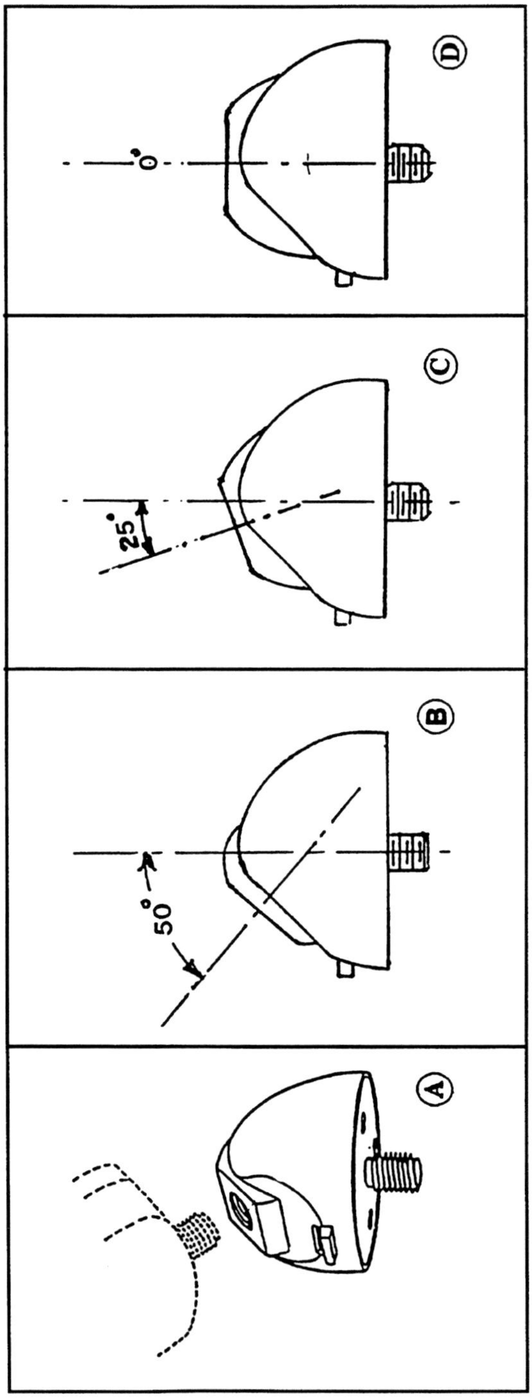


Figure 68. A wrist flexion unit. (A) Terminal device is connected to the movable part of the flexion unit. (B,C, & D) Detents hold the terminal device in 50, 25, or 0 degree position.

## Elbow Units

All transhumeral, elbow-disarticulation, and some transradial amputees require an elbow joint if the prosthesis is to be functional.

### *Elbows for Transhumeral and Shoulder Disarticulation Amputees*

The classical unit for transhumeral amputees permits active flexion about the elbow while depending on gravity for extension. An alternating lock, in which the same small linear motion that is used to lock the elbow in a desired position also unlocks the elbow upon the next

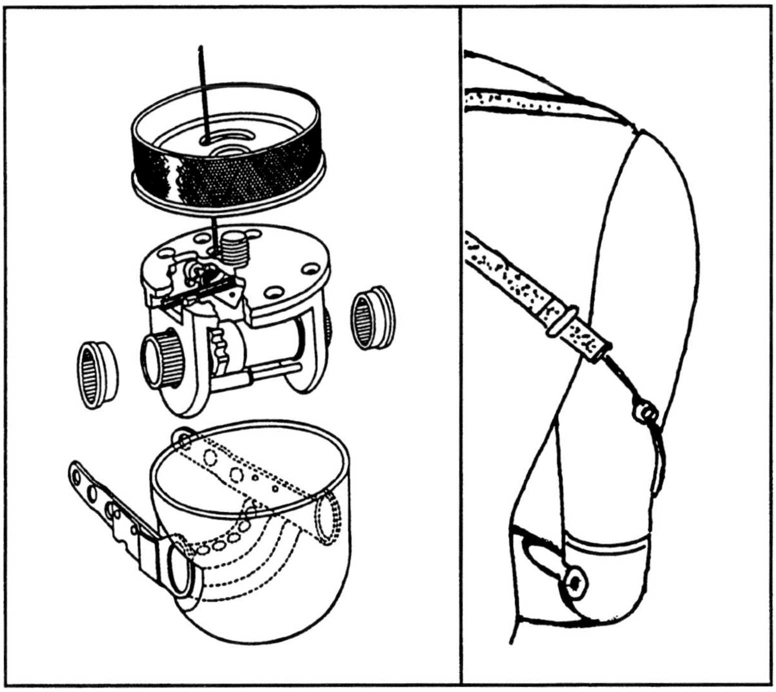

Figure 69. Elbow unit for transhumeral and shoulder disarticulation amputees. Tension on the control cable alternately locks and unlocks the elbow in any of eleven positions of flexion. Left drawing, courtesy of *Artificial Limbs.*

activation, is the current standard (Figure 69). The elbow is attached to the humeral section of the artificial arm by a turntable that permits manual control of rotation about the long axis of the humeral section. When in the extended position, the forearm is allowed to swing freely.

To reduce the force required to flex the elbow, a small adjustable coil spring assembly, or lift assist unit, can be added to the exterior of the elbow, usually on the medial side. The spring can be adjusted so that it is just sufficiently strong to be of assistance but not so strong that it will keep the forearm from assuming the extended position as a consequence of gravity. The lift-assist unit may be added or removed without affecting the mechanism of the elbow unit itself. Alternating locking elbows are available in a range of sizes including at least one suitable for children.

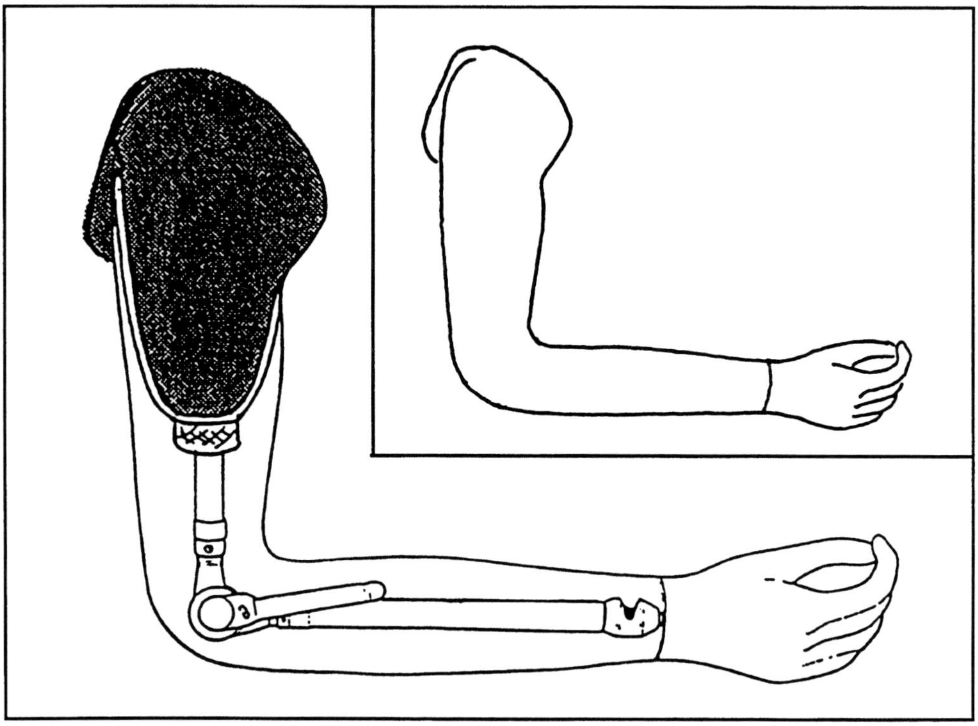

Figure 70. Schematic of a passive prosthesis for a transhumeral amputees. Elbow flexion and humeral rotation may be adjusted by the contralateral arm. The position is maintained by friction.

For passive arms, a relatively simple elbow that can be positioned and adjusted manually in two planes, elbow flexion-extension and humeral rotation, is available (Figure 70). The lock is activated manually by application of force to the locking lever through the soft foam cover. Friction in the joints maintains the position selected until a change is desired.

### *Elbows for Elbow Disarticulation Amputees*

In the elbow disarticulation case, the space usually occupied by the artificial elbow unit designed for transhumeral amputees is not available. Location of such units distal to the stump is not only unsightly, but does not allow for the terminal device to be operated close to the face. To solve this problem, metal hinges with a locking mechanism that can be installed on the outside of the socket are available (Figure 71). The compromise that has to be made is that these units are not as strong as those intended for higher levels, and manual rotation about the long axis of the humerus cannot be provided, and thus making close attention necessary for optimum location of the hinges, but the advantages of an elbow disarticulation stump far outweigh these disadvantages. Outside locking elbow units are available in "large," "medium," and "small" sizes. The largest size is also available in a "heavy-duty" model.

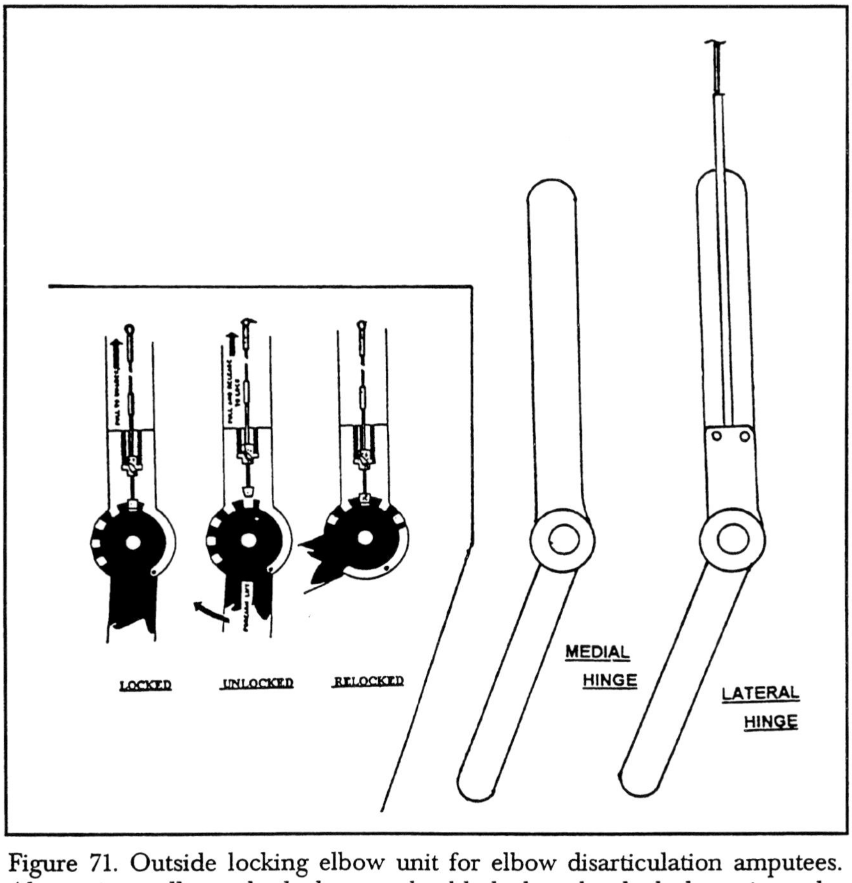


Figure 71. Outside locking elbow unit for elbow disarticulation amputees. Alternating pulls on the lock control cable lock and unlock the unit on the medial side. Five positions of flexion are provided. Insert, courtesy of *Artificial Limbs.*

### *Elbow Units for Transradial Amputees*

Typical methods of fitting long and medium length transradial stumps are shown in Figure 72. For the amputee who is not engaged in heavy manual activities, flexible hinges are used as elbow "joints" to take advantage of the residual pronation and supination. These hinges may be of leather or a flexible metal cable which is available with special end fittings designed for one end to be laminated into the socket wall.

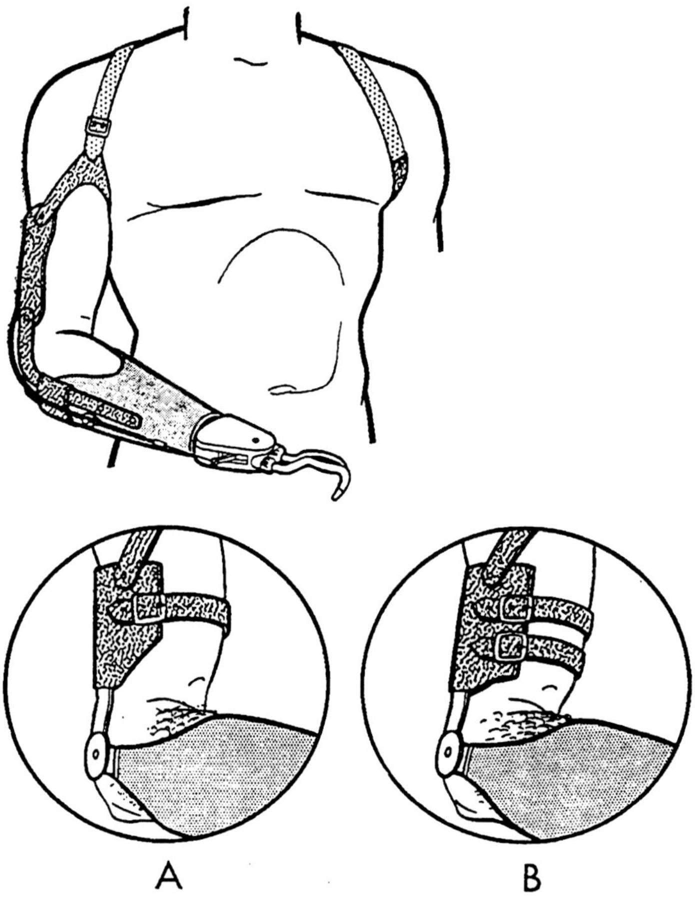


Figure 72. Typical methods for fitting medium to long transradial stumps. Where possible an open cuff and flexible hinges are used. When more stability between socket and stump is required rigid hinges and closed cuffs can be used (inserts A and B). Courtesy of *Artificial Limbs.*

For the amputee who will be performing heavy manual labor simple, single-axis metal hinges can be used (Inserts a and b, Figure 72) to provide more stability between socket and stump. A polycentric version is available to reduce as much as possible relative motion between the patient and prosthesis, but it is not as strong. Obviously, one of the disadvantages of the use of rigid hinges is the restriction of rotation of the forearm stump.

Before the introduction of the self-suspending socket for short and very short transradial stumps, a host of elbow units was developed to take advantage of whatever function these abbreviated stumps offered. At least three of these designs are still available, and are shown in Figure 73, since occasionally they are useful in solving an individual problem when the self-suspending socket is contraindicated.

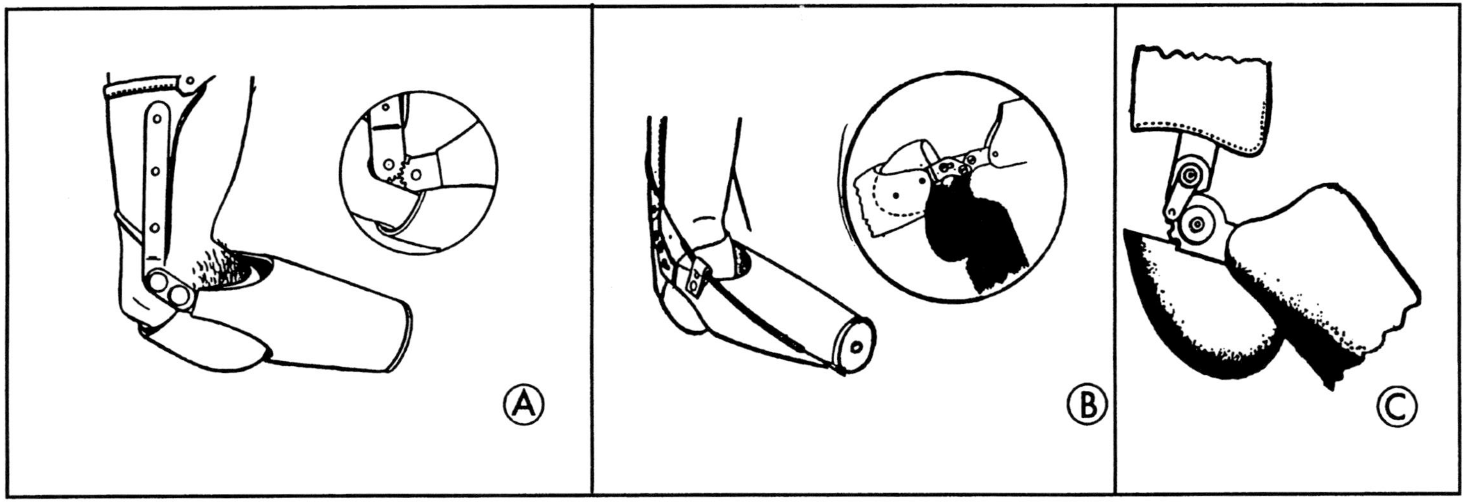


Figure 73. Elbow units designed for short and very short transradial cases. These units are seldom used today, but are available and can be used occasionally for very special cases. (A) Geared step-up hinges that give a 2:1 ratio between movement of the artificial forearm and the stump. Available in small, medium, and large sizes. (B) Sliding action step-up hinge that provides less than a 2:1 ratio and thus protrudes less. (C) Stump-activated locking elbow unit for very short transradial amputees. Shoulder harnessing is used to provide elbow flexion, and the lock is controlled by movement of the stump in extension and flexion. Courtesy of Artificial Limbs

For the short stump that cannot provide the range of elbow flexion desired, "step-up" hinges which amplify the range of motion may be prescribed. Two types are available (Figure 73). One design doubles the flexion range by means of gears; the other known as the "variable ratio" or "sliding action" hinge (Figure 73) produces essentially the same results but reduces the amount of protrusion of the stump and socket in the fully flexed position. It is often necessary to use a "dual" harness system to provide the necessary force for elbow flexion, because the effective torque about the artificial elbow is halved as a result of the 2:1 increase in elbow flexion.

When the stump is too short to provide enough flexion to take advantage of step-up hinges, it can be used to lock and unlock outside elbow locking elbow hinges (Figure 73).

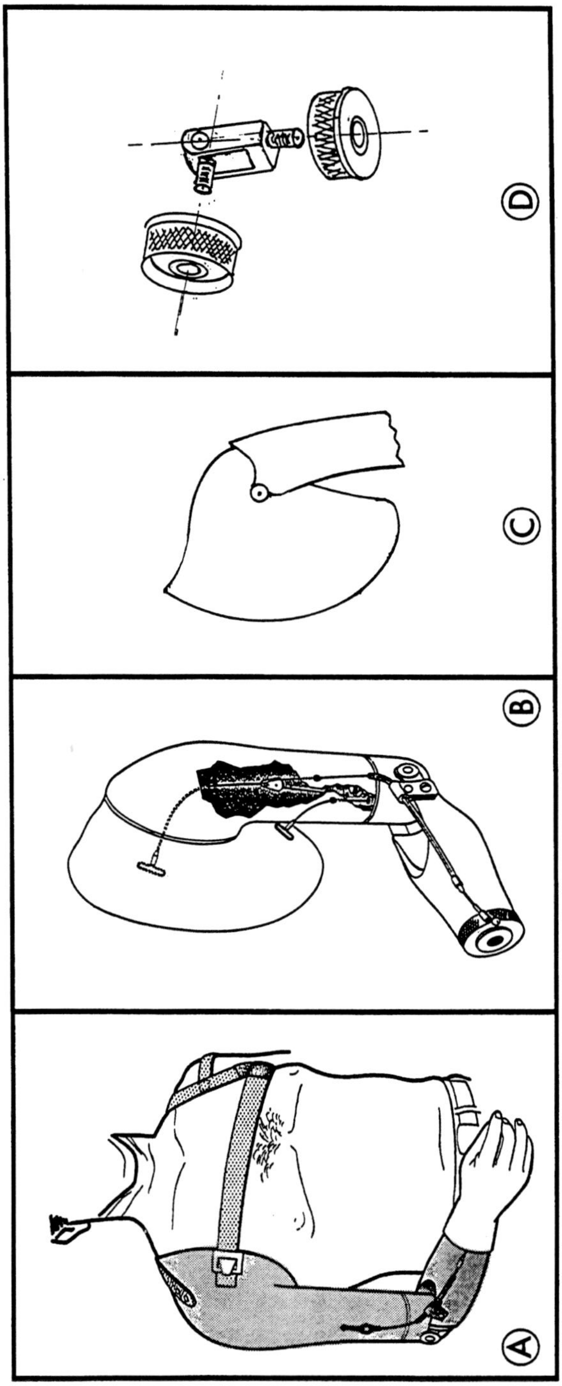


Figure 74. Shoulder joints. (A) Joint integral with socket and arm section, used when a segment of the humerus remains. This type of prosthesis is the most stable of all for amputations about the elbow. Courtesy of Artificial Limbs. (B) Bulkhead joint installed in the sagittal plane. Arm position can be held in place by friction between the two plates. Courtesy of Artificial Limbs. (C) Single-axis joint can allow freedom for abduction of shoulder joint to make donning clothes somewhat easier. (D) A combination of wrist units can make manual positioning in abduction and flexion at the same time.

### Shoulder Units

Unfortunately, there are no functional shoulder joints for shoulder disarticulation and forequarter disarticulation amputees. Several types of connections are available to permit manual adjustment of the position of the humeral section with respect to the socket (Figure 74). Shoulder "bulkheads" permit flexion and extension, approximately in the sagittal plane. When adjustment is desired in the abduction-adduction plane, also, a "two-way," or "shoulder flexion abduction," joint is used. Motion in three planes can be had with use of the "universal shoulder joint" which uses two standard wrist friction units coupled by a threaded single axis hinge (Figure 74D).

### Harness Systems

The common method for operation of upper-limb, body-powered prostheses is use of a harness about the shoulders to transmit the force and excursion generated by relative motion between segments of the body (21,48). In most cases, however, the harness is also used to help keep the prosthesis in place. Harnesses are generally made of one-inch wide Dacron webbing, or straps, and a Bowden cable with specially designed fittings is used for the power transmission system (Figure 60).

Patterns based on sound physiological and biomechanical principles that permit clever and efficient use of the limited power and excursion available have been developed through the years and appear to have reached the zenith of development. Unfortunately, comfort is difficult to obtain especially in the case of the unilateral amputee, and no improvement seems to be in sight. Still, the use of a harness provides the highest quality of sensory feedback yet devised.

Harness systems vary with respect to the level of amputation and the energy sources available, and whether or not the amputee is expected to engage in hard labor. Ironically, the more functions that need replacement, the less power in the form of force and excursion for activation and control of the substitute devices is available.

The three major sources of force and excursion for operation and control of upper-limb body-powered prostheses are biscapular abduction, shoulder flexion, and arm extension (Figure 59). The Bowden cable permits fairly efficient transmission of force and excursion between two points that move with respect to each other.

When no suspensory function is required of the harness, i.e., wrist disarticulation cases, a simple loop about the axilla region on the contralateral side usually suffices. Relative motion between the axilla and the upper arm as the shoulder is flexed provides the power for control of the terminal device.

When suspension is required and the amputee is not expected to engage in strenuous activities, a "figure-eight" harness is used (Figure 75). In the typical transradial case the strap that passes over the axilla area is crossed over itself near the centerline of the body, and the strap that starts off as the lower one is passed over the shoulder on the amputated side and fastened to the socket through a triceps pad or humeral cuff. A Bowden cable is attached to the other end of the strap and its reaction point is attached to the posterior aspect of the triceps pad or humeral cuff.

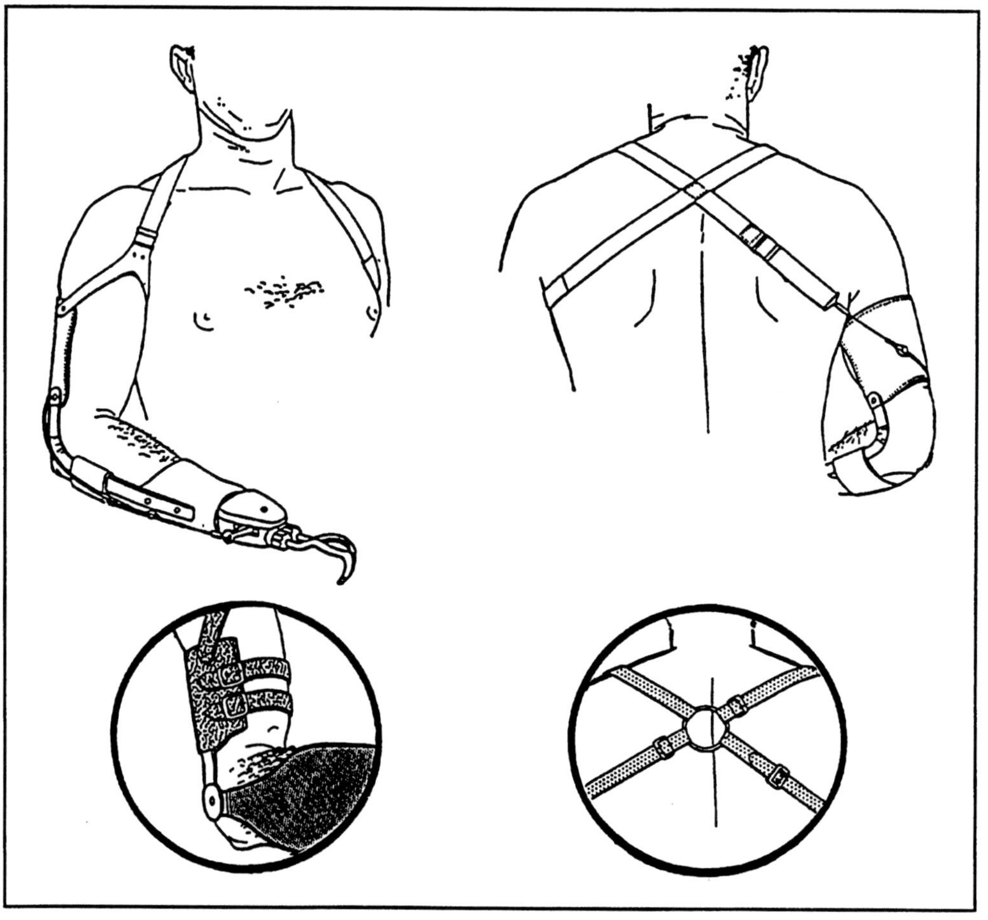

Figure 75. Figure-8 harness applied to a transradial case. Shown in the bottom, left, insert is a biceps cuff and single-axis metal hinges used when strenuous activity is expected. Shown in the bottom, right, insert is the ring-type harness used instead of sewing the harness at the crossover point. Selection is usually based on the physical characteristics of the patient. Modified from *Artificial Limbs.*

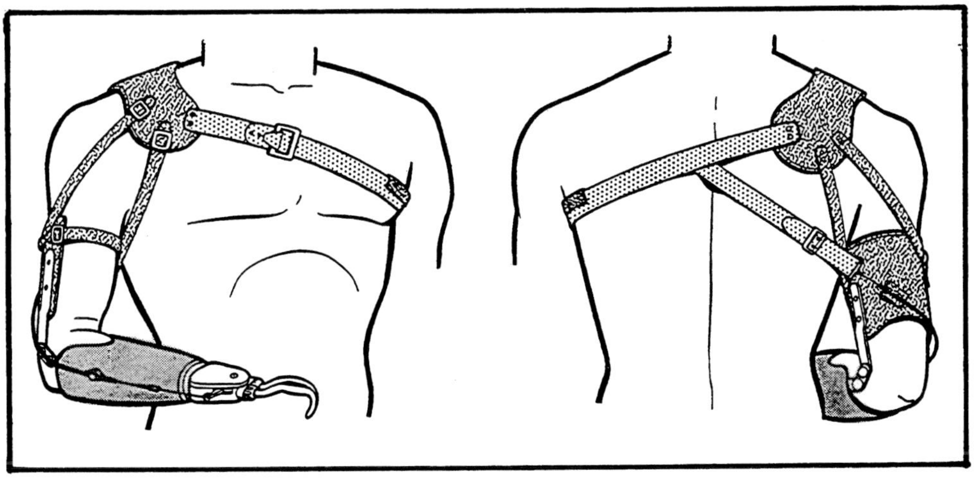

Figure 76. The transradial chest strap harness. The two suspension straps running through D-rings are attached to a leather shoulder saddle. Improved stability and reduced unit stresses over the shoulder offer greater ability to lift axial loads. Normally, a half-cuff and rigid elbow hinges are used with the transradial chest strap harness. Courtesy of *Artificial Limbs.*

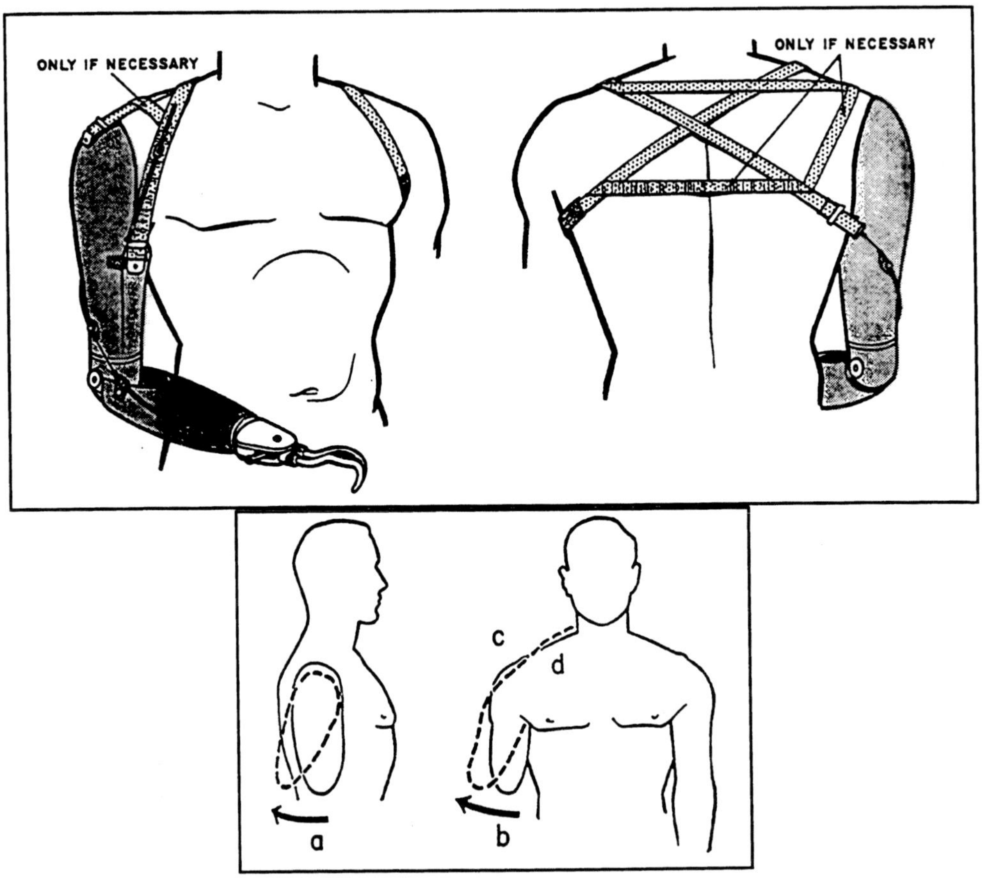


Figure. 77. *Upper*, The transhumeral figure-8 harness. The basic structure consists of a loop about the axilla on the unaffected side, the front portion supporting the socket and the rear portion attaching to the control cable so that relative motion between the torso and the stump can be used to control both elbow flexion and terminal device operation. The Bowden cable is split so that tension in the cable causes the forearm to lift when the artificial elbow is unlocked and permits terminal device operation when it is locked. *Lower*, Sketch showing the coordinated motions usually used to lock and unlock the elbow unit. At the same time the stump is both extended (a) and abducted (b) while the shoulder is depressed (c) and the trapezius is bulged (d) by downward rotation of the scapula. Courtesy of *Artificial Limbs.*

When the transradial amputee is expected to engage in heavy manual labor or other strenuous activity, the chest-strap harness (Figure 76) is usually used. A "saddle" over the shoulder on the amputated side helps suspend the prosthesis. The improved stability and lower unit pressures in the axilla area due to the saddle increase the ability to lift axial loads. A half-cuff and rigid elbow hinges are usually used to provide an optimum degree of stability between amputee and socket.

In the typical transhumeral case, the end of the harness that is passed over the shoulder on the amputated side is fastened to the anterior aspect of the socket, and the Bowden cable fitting is fastened on the lateral aspect of the socket (Figure 77). The control system used almost universally in the U.S. for transhumeral amputees is the "dual control" harness, in which the excursion generated in the control cable is used not only for operation of the terminal device but for flexion of the elbow as well. For this to work, the Bowden cable housing must be split between the two fittings. When the desired amount of elbow flexion is reached, the elbow is locked and the force is transmitted to the terminal device. The drawback here is that the excursion available must be divided between the two functions.

In certain areas of Europe, the so-called triple control harness is used so as to eliminate the need for locking the elbow and thus have more excursion available for each function, but the harnessing is complex and a great deal of time is generally required to acquire the skills required to use it properly.

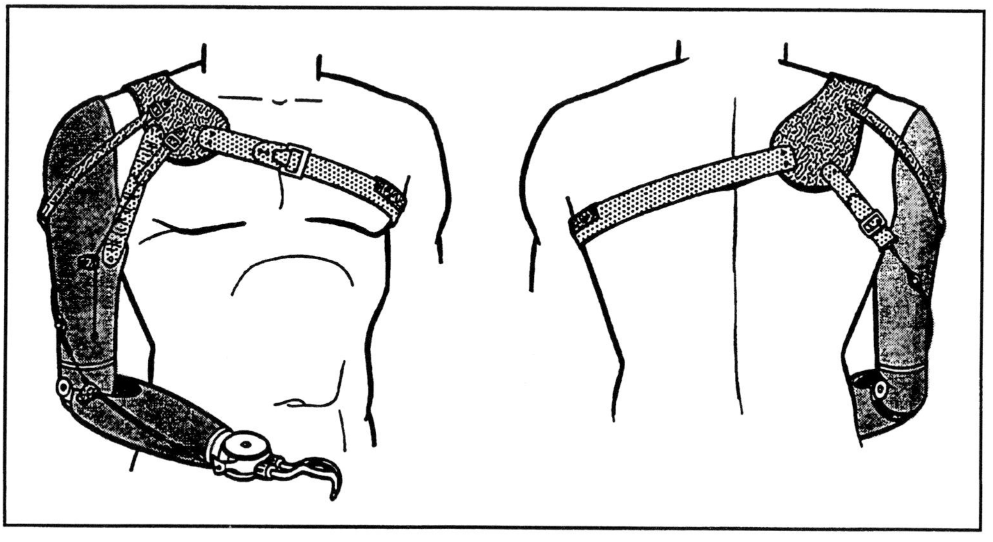

Fig. 78. Chest strap harness for transhumeral amputations. Use of the chest strap and shoulder saddle reduces unit pressures over the shoulder and axilla, but restricts motion somewhat. It is used when relatively heavy labor or other strenuous activity is anticipated. Courtesy of *Artificial Limbs.*

When strenuous activity is expected to be the norm the "chest strap" harness is used (Figure 78). A flexible, usually leather, shoulder saddle is located over the shoulder on the affected side. A fairly wide strap with an adjustable buckle is passed around the chest under the axilla to hold the saddle in place with respect to the contralateral side of the torso. Two or more straps from the shoulder saddle to the proximal portion of the socket help hold it in place. This arrangement provides for lower unit pressures over the shoulder and in the axilla area as well as increased stability needed for strenuous activities, but obviously it is more restrictive of movement.

Harness patterns for shoulder and forequarter disarticulations are based on the principles set forth here, but the prosthetist has a much more limited source of excursion and force for use in meeting a greater loss of function than cases at lower levels.

## Prescription of Body-Powered Prosthesis

The first consideration in prescription of body-powered prostheses is almost universally the specific type of terminal device that the amputee will use most of the time. After that comes the selection of the other components based on the sources and amount of power available. The harness pattern usually evolves simultaneously with the selection of the components. In providing a prescription, it is important to remember that there should be a minimum of restriction, if any, to the movement and thus function of all residual motion in the limbs and body, and that each of these motions has potential for either providing a function itself or activating and controlling a function.

### Prostheses for Partial Hand Amputations

Because surgeons make every effort to salvage whatever function possible in treating hands subjected to trauma, there are no established patterns of results. Each result is unique, and prosthetics treatment for each case is unique if maximum return of function is to be achieved (6). Consequently, virtually no off-the-shelf components are available, and the prosthetist must improvise. Some innovative solutions that have been used in the past are shown in Figure 79. Nearly all seek to achieve some form of prehension, often by providing a rigid apposition "post."

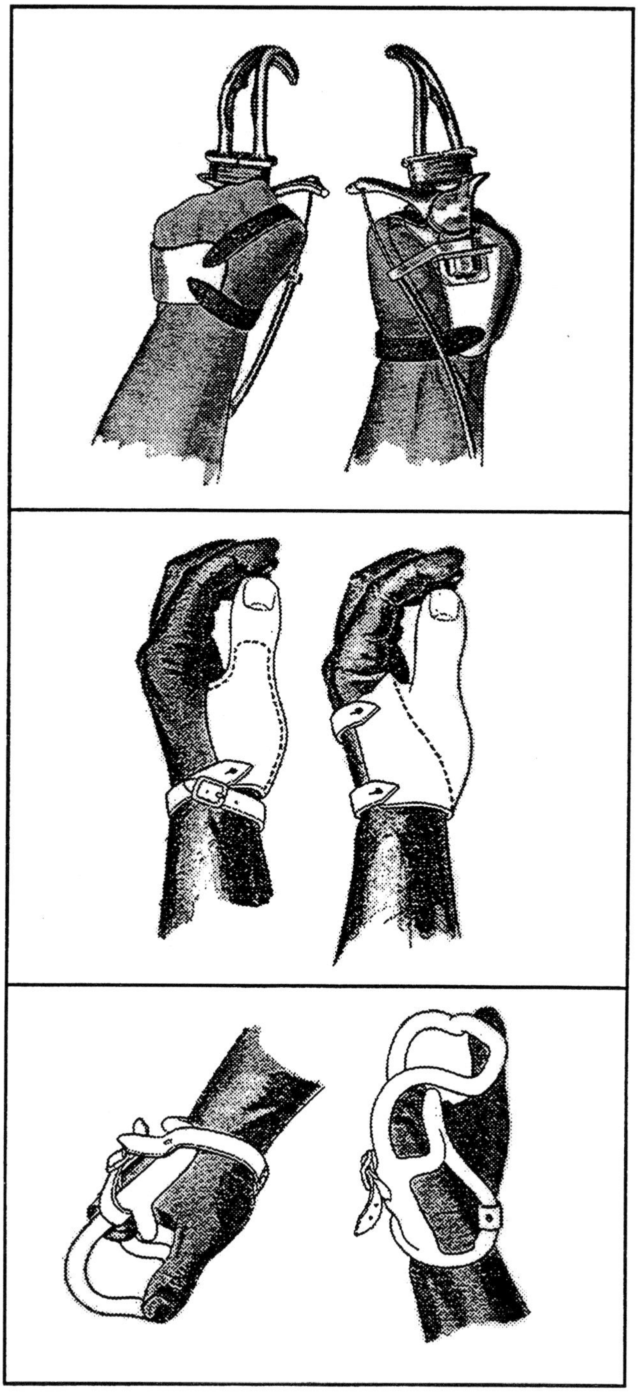

Figure 79. Three examples of augmentation of function for partial hand amputations. Courtesy of *Artificial Limbs.*

## Prostheses for the Wrist Disarticulation Amputee

Usually the wrist disarticulation stump is capable of about two-thirds of the 180 degree range of supination-pronation usually found in an intact limb. Any socket will impose some restriction on this function, but the restriction can be kept to a minimum if the socket is fitted a bit loose and trimmed as shown in Figure 80. The length of the stump makes it necessary to use one of the wrist units designed especially for this level of amputation. The quick change feature often has to be sacrificed for a more anthropomorphic arrangement and better cosmesis. Because of the many functions unaffected by amputation at the wrist, harnessing for the wrist disarticulation amputee is not complicated, consisting normally of a simple figure-eight system. A triceps pad and long, flexible hinges are usually required to route the Bowden cable properly.

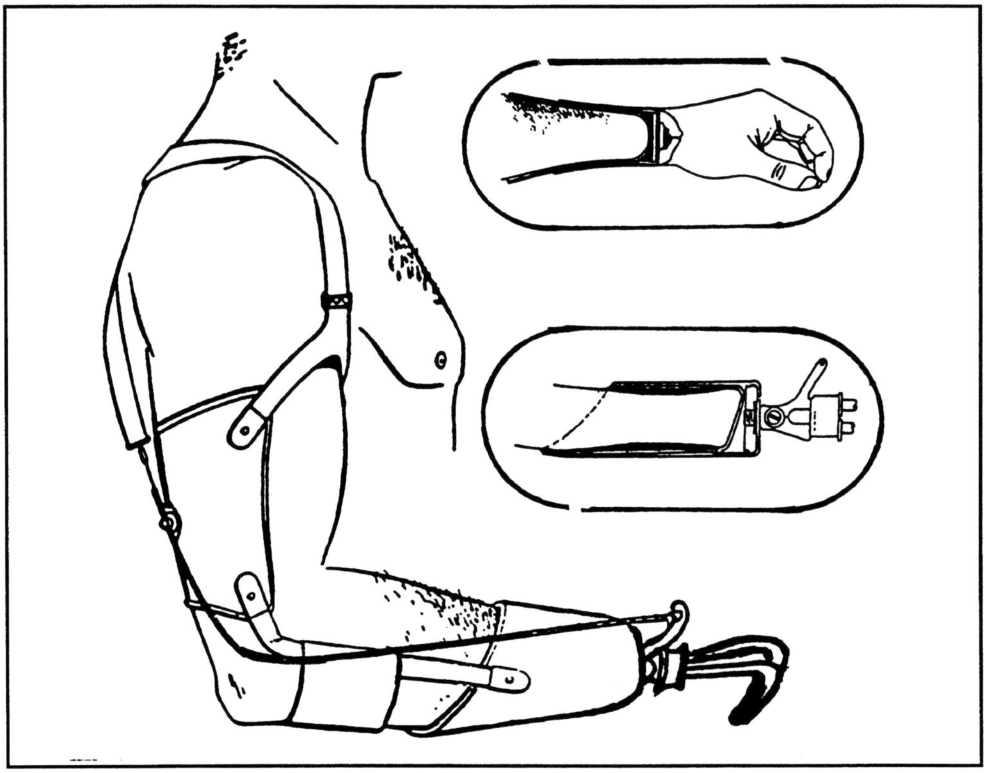

Figure 80. Typical fitting for a wrist disarticulation case. Insets show two methods of attaching terminal devices. In the upper inset, the stud of the terminal device is replaced by a fitting that can be laminated into the socket, thereby providing a prosthesis commensurate with the normal limb. A separate socket must be provided if the amputee is to interchange terminal devices. The very short wrist unit shown in the lower insert is more common. Modified from *Artificial Limbs.*

## Prostheses for Transradial Amputees

Because residual function of the transradial stump is affected adversely as the level of amputation moves toward the elbow, transradial stumps have been divided into four distinct groups: *long, medium, short,* and *very short* (Figure 81). Hardware and harness patterns are available to take advantage of the functions that remain in each instance.

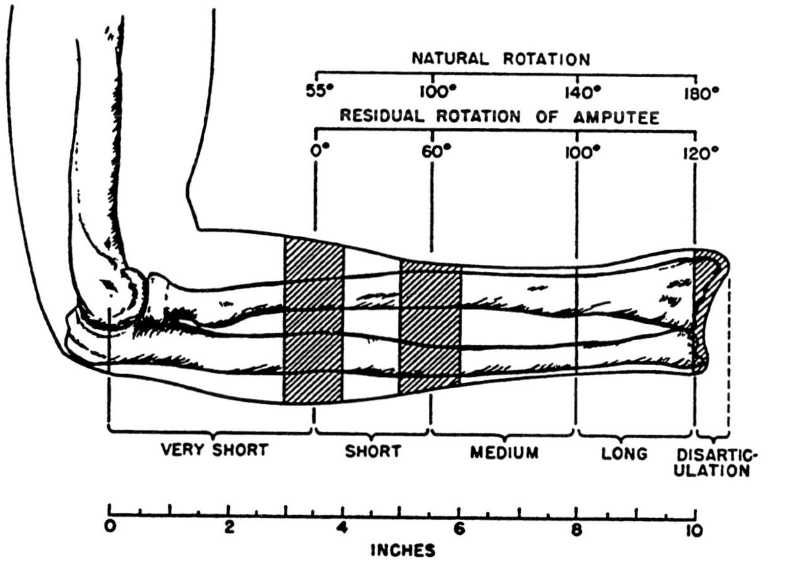


Figure 81. Schematic showing the amount of pronation-supination remaining in a transradial amputation with respect to length. Also shown is a classification of transradial amputation stumps according to length. From (55).

### *Prostheses for Long Transradial Amputees*

For long transradial amputees the prosthesis is much the same as that for the wrist disarticulation case except that longer and stronger wrist units can be used (Figure 77). The fit of the socket trim of the proximal border is such that as much as possible of the residual rotation of the stump is allowed while maintaining an intimate relationship between socket and stump. Harnessing is commensurate with the use expected.

### *Prostheses for Medium Transradial Amputees*

The same dictum applies in the case of medium length trans-radial stumps (Figure 77), but the harness will be asked to provide more of a suspensory function than is the case with longer stumps. Rigid hinges and a humeral cuff may be required to provide the stability and suspension required (Figure 75). Rigid hinges, of course, preclude active pronation and supination of the forearm.

### *Prostheses for Short Transradial Stumps*

It is often difficult to fit the short transradial amputee so as to obtain a full range of flexion about the elbow. "Step-up" hinges (Figure 73) that amplify elbow flexion can be used, but it is more common to use one of the "self-suspending" socket designs proposed originally by a group in Muenster, Germany and modified by others (Figure 82). In

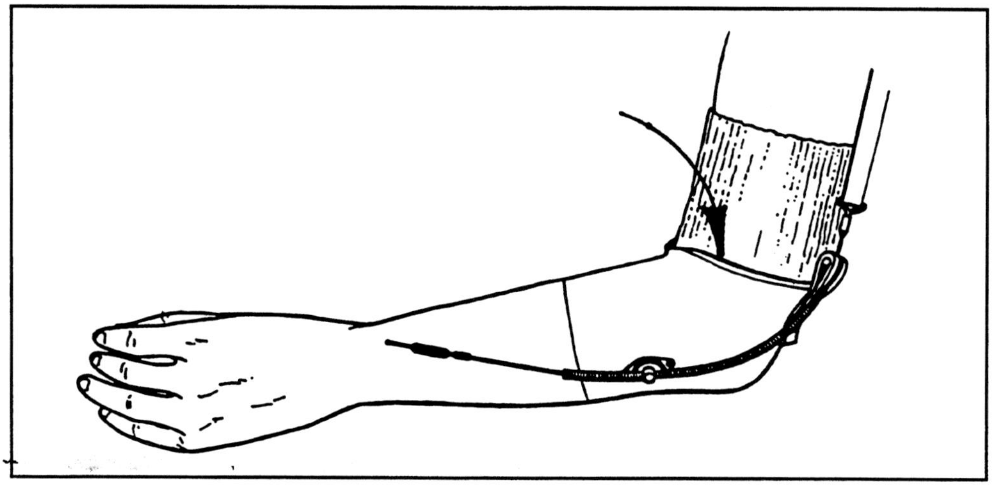

Figure 82. The Muenster-type socket for the short transradial amputee. The anterior trim line is brought to the crease between the arm and forearm to avoid the bunching of soft tissues as the elbow is flexed. While this arrangement normally restricts the range of elbow flexion, this can be compensated for by building in 10-30 degrees of initial flexion in the socket.

the self-suspending socket, the brim is extended above the epicondyles of the humerus to hold the socket in place. This, of course, restricts flexion somewhat, but not to the degree that would be expected if the socket trim line were extended to the fold of the arm and forearm on the anterior aspect of the stump so that the soft tissues are not allowed to bunch as the elbow is flexed.. Some of the loss of flexion can be compensated for by incorporating 10 to 30 degrees of "flexion" in the forearm-socket. This amount of "preflexion" usually goes unnoticed by casual observers since the elbow is seldom carried fully extended, but permits the amputee to use the terminal device in the vicinity of the face and head without the need for complicated mechanical contrivances.

A distinct advantage of the "self-suspending" socket is that the simplest of harnessing systems is required.

### *Prostheses for Very Short Transradial Amputations*

When the stump of a transradial amputation is so short that the Muenster technique will not work, the stump can be used to activate outside locking elbow hinges normally used for elbow disarticulation cases, thus simplifying the harnessing that would be required otherwise (Figure 73C).

## Prostheses for Transhumeral Amputations

For operation of the terminal device, in most instances the elbow must be in the locked position. The alternating lock feature of the elbow units available permits the elbow to be locked and unlocked easily by a small amount of relative motion between the shoulder and prosthesis (Figure 69). The excursion required is so small that the motion is hardly noticed. The friction of the turntable of the elbow can be adjusted so that the amputee can rotate the forearm about the long axis of the humerus with the contralateral limb, artificial or normal, or by pushing against a stationary object to position as desired. Passive wrist flexion units can be prescribed as warranted. If the amputee expects to use hand and hook interchangeably, one of the quick-change wrist units (Figure 67) should be prescribed.

There are many variations in the design of sockets for the transhumeral amputation, and indications for prescription are not clear. Most of the differences are in the trim of the proximal border of the socket. Suction, or pressure differential, for suspension (47) has been found to be desirable by many prosthetists and amputees.

## Prostheses for Elbow Disarticulation Amputees

The principles of prostheses for the transhumeral amputee apply equally as well to the elbow disarticulation amputee, except that the elbow joint is installed on the outside of the socket (Figure 83). Harnessing is essentially the same. The socket usually contains an elastic liner to provide a snug fit around and above the epicondyles, making suspension of the prosthesis, and to some degree harnessing, less of a problem than when amputation is at higher levels. The one disadvantage to this system is the lack of a means of prepositioning the forearm about the long axis of the humerus.

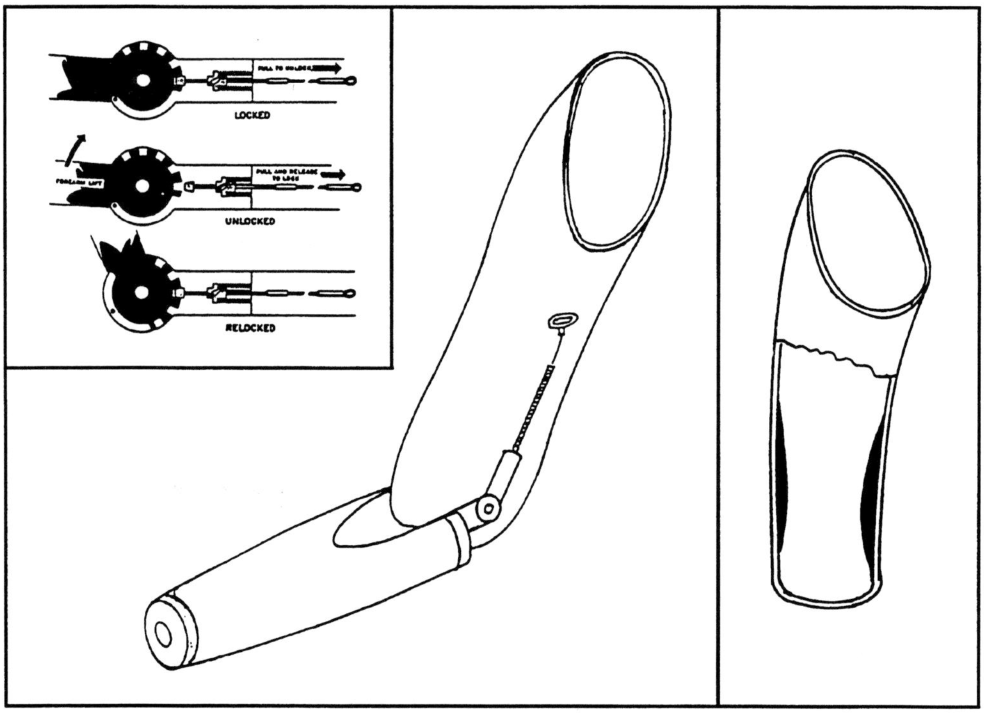


Figure 83. Typical socket and elbow unit for an elbow disarticulation prosthesis. The inset on the left shows the action of the alternating locking elbow unit. The illustration on the right shows the shape of the socket when an elastomer is used to allow entry into the socket while at the same time providing some degree of suspension.

## Prostheses for Shoulder Disarticulation and Forequarter Amputees

Provision of a functional prosthesis for shoulder and forequarter disarticulation amputees presents a most difficult problem to prosthetists and designers. Not only is there more function lost than in the transhumeral case (Figure 84), but there is less force and excursion available for activation and control. The typical shoulder disarticulation prosthesis uses one of the several passive shoulder joints available (Figure 74). A "nudge" control (Figure 85) can be used for locking and unlocking the elbow when the more conventional methods fail. The nudge control is usually located on the anterior aspect of the socket so that movement of the neck and chin provides the force and excursion to activate the locking mechanism in the elbow originally designed for the transhumeral amputee.

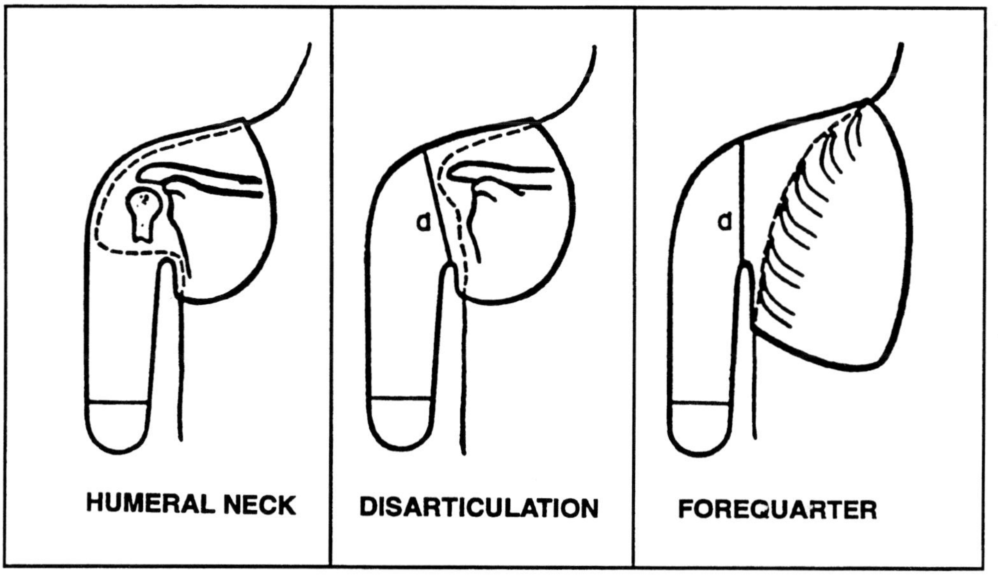


Figure 84. Schematics of shoulder sockets. Solid lines show residual bony structure; dashed lines, the body contour and inner wall of the socket. Disarticulation at the shoulder and forequarter may be two-piece with sectional plates (a) or joints (Fig. 74). Courtesy *Artificial Limbs.*

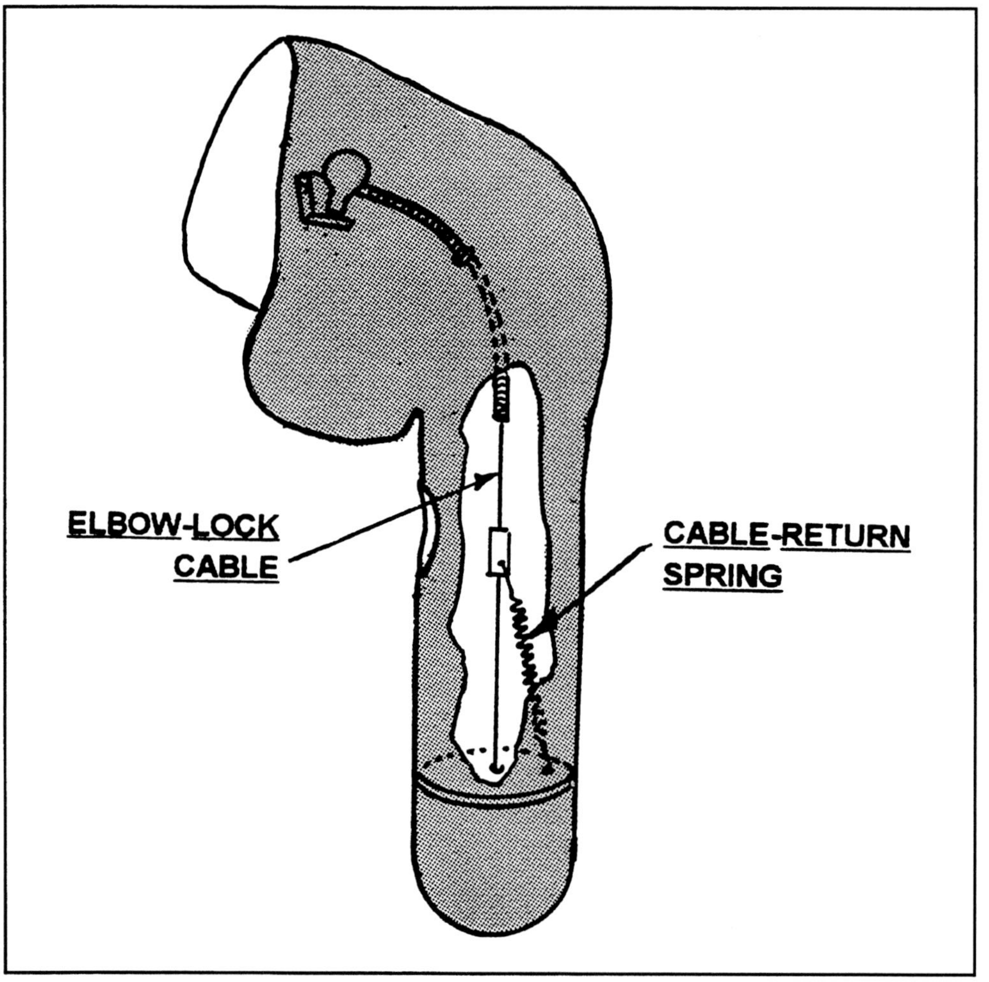


Figure 85. Nudge control for for locking and unlocking an elbow unit. The nudge control is usually mounted on the anterior aspect of the socket so that it can be activated by the chin.

The socket for the shoulder disarticulation case may cover the shoulder entirely or may be of the "frame," or fenestrated, type (Figure 86) where a portion of the chest may be exposed to avoid excessive heat build-up. The harness is usually of the chest strap type.

Prostheses for the forequarter amputee are essentially the same as for the shoulder disarticulation case. Stabilization of the socket is, of course, more difficult. Because of the almost insurmountable difficulties in providing a functional prosthesis for the forequarter amputee, the most common practice at this time is to provide a lightweight cap to fill the void left by the amputation so that the patient can wear clothes that do not require alteration.

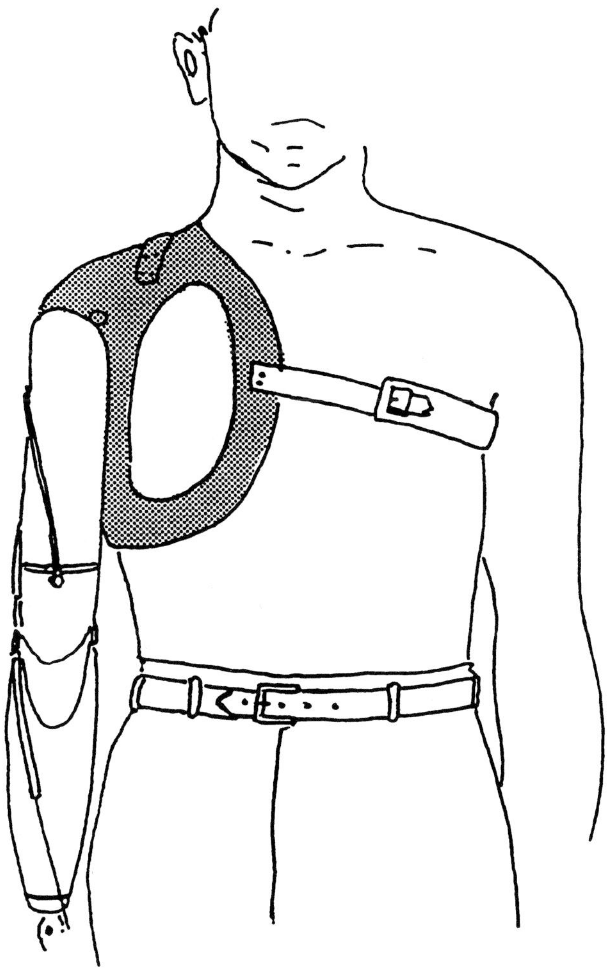

Figure 86. Fenestrated socket for the shoulder disarticulation amputee when perspiration or elevated temperature is a problem.

## Prostheses for Bilateral Upper-Limb Amputees

Except for bilateral cases involving shoulder disarticulation and forequarter amputation, fitting the bilateral upper limb amputee presents few problems that are not encountered with the unilateral case. The prostheses used are generally the same as those prescribed for corresponding levels in unilateral cases. Artificial hands are rarely used by bilateral amputees, because hooks afford so much more function. Most bilateral cases find that the wrist-flexion unit, at least on one side, is quite useful.

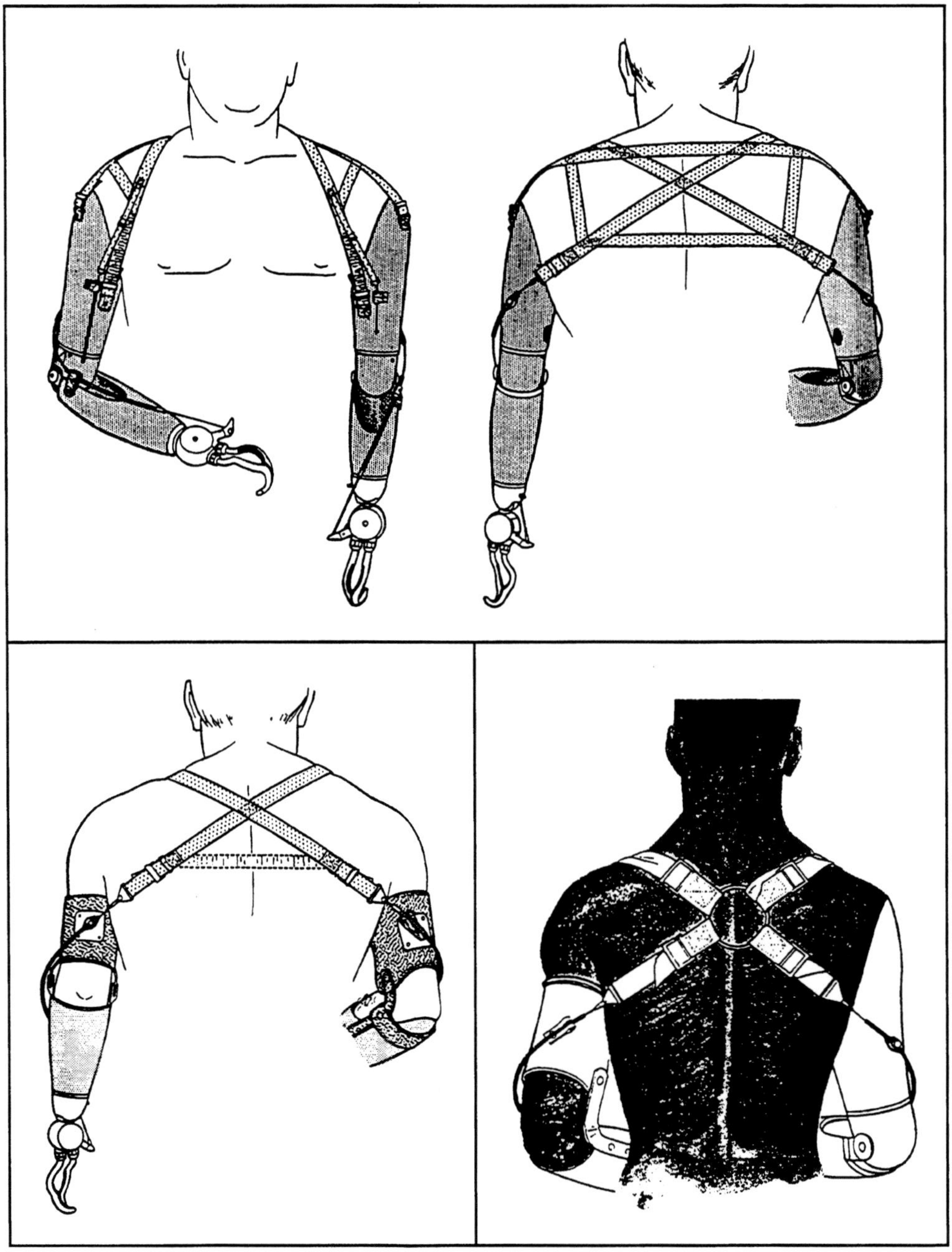

Figure 87. Typical harnessing for bilateral upper limb amputees. Top, bilateral transhumeral case; Lower left, bilateral transradial case; Lower right, one transradial and one transhumeral. Courtesy of *Artificial Limbs*.

The harness for each prosthesis may be separated, but it is general practice to combine the two (Figure 87). Because the reaction forces in the control system against the body are spread over a larger area of the body than is the case in the unilateral case, the coupled bilateral system is probably considerably the more comfortable of the two. Furthermore, when the two harnesses are combined, it is easier for the amputee to don the prostheses unaided.

Some prosthetists have claimed success in fitting bilateral shoulder-disarticulation cases with two functional prostheses. Because of the lack of sufficient sources of energy for control, most cases of this type are provided with a functional prosthesis on one side and a plastic cap over the opposite shoulder to provide an anchor for the harness. It seems logical that externally-powered prostheses would be most useful here, but lack of control sites presents the same problem found in body-powered prostheses.

## EXTERNALLY-POWERED PROSTHESES

An obvious way to solve many of the problems of restoring function to the upper-limb amputee would seem to be use of electrical power. With the availability of very small but powerful batteries and motors, it has been possible to devise prostheses that provide the power necessary to operate upper limb prostheses at acceptable functional and cosmetic levels. Some amputees find electrically-powered prostheses useful enough that they are worn continuously, in spite of the lack of sensory feedback that is as acute as that commonly found in body-powered, or harness-controlled, prostheses. For amputations at levels above the elbow, it is possible to use electricity to power elbow and wrist units, and use a harness to activate and control a terminal device, and thus retain the sensory feedback offered by a body harness.

### Components Available

Competition in the development and manufacture of components for electrical prostheses is keen and there is available a sizable armamentarium to choose from in preparation of a prescription (7,23,33,39,59). Available components can be classified into three main groups: *hand substitutes*, or prehensors, *wrist units*, and *elbows*. Electrically-actuated locks for cable-controlled elbow units are also available, but as yet there are no electrically-actuated shoulder units.

Anthropomorphic electric hands are available, and are perhaps the most used terminal devices, especially in transradial cases (Figure 88). When there is room to store batteries in the distal part of the forearm and a "Muenster" type socket with electrodes installed in the socket walls is used the result is a self-contained prosthesis that requires no harness. At least one electrically-operated hook (Figure 89) is available and the Otto Bock firm offers a "Greifer" (gripper) (Figure 90) in which the jaws are parallel in all positions and provision for manual operation of wrist flexion is built in. Electrically-powered wrist units that provide pronation and supination are also available.

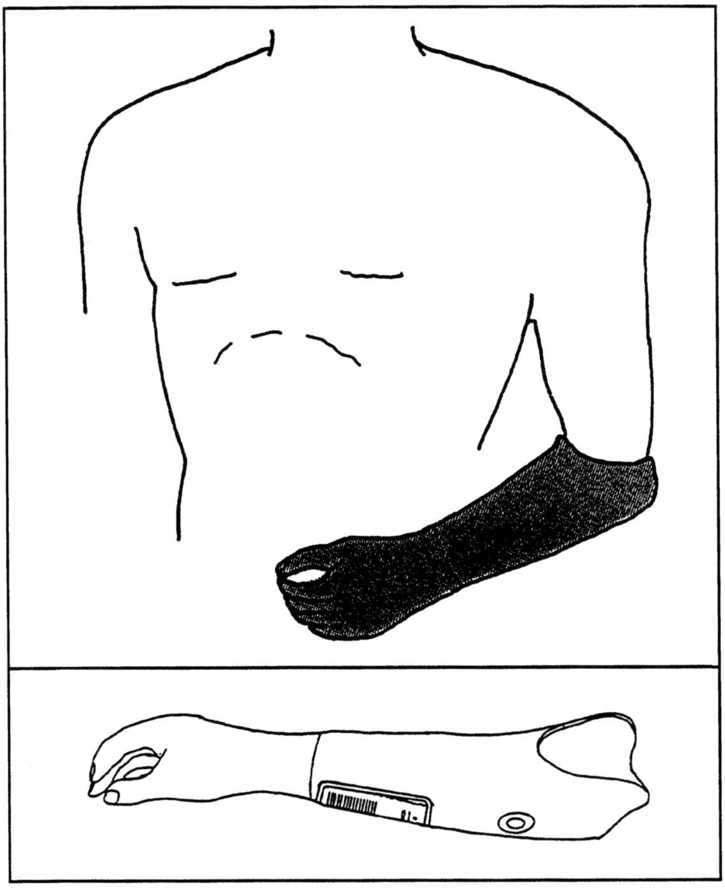

Figure 88. Typical transradial myoelectric prosthesis. The motor is located just proximal to the terminal device and wrist unit, and the small, thin battery is usually attached to the exterior wallof the forearm. Electrodes are embedded in the socket wall. An electrically operated wrist rotation unit is an option.

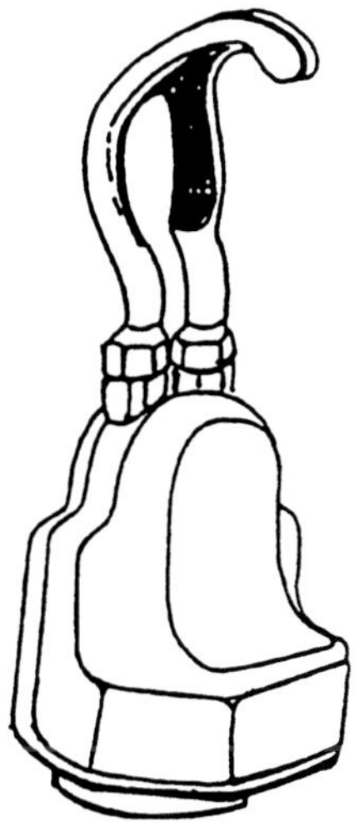

Figure 89. An electrically powered hook-type terminal device.

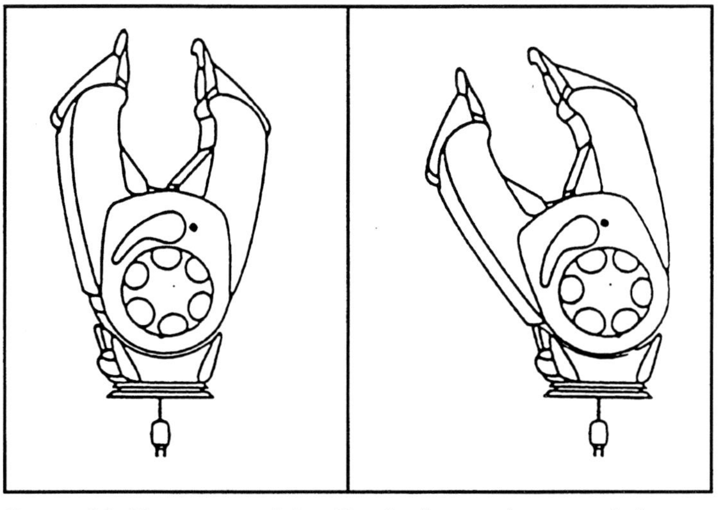

Figure 90. Two views of the Greifer (gripper) terminal device. The "jaws" are parallel to each other at all times. The wrist flexion function is controlled manually. Courtesy of Otto Bock Orthopedic Industries.

Conventional terminal devices can be used by transhumeral amputees by installing a prehension actuator" (Figure 91), a forearm unit that contains an electric motor and battery that provides linear motion to a cable with standard fittings for connection to a standard terminal device. The prehension actuator may be controlled by either a mechanical switch or a myoelectric signal.

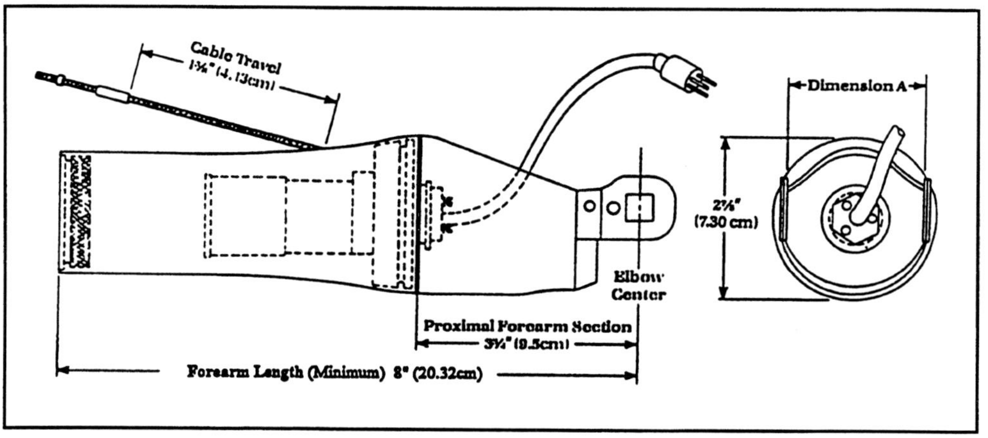


Figure 91. Side view of the prehensor device. The rotary motion of an electric motor is converted to linear motion (cable travel) for operation of a conventional terminal device. Courtesy of Hosmer Dorrance Corp.

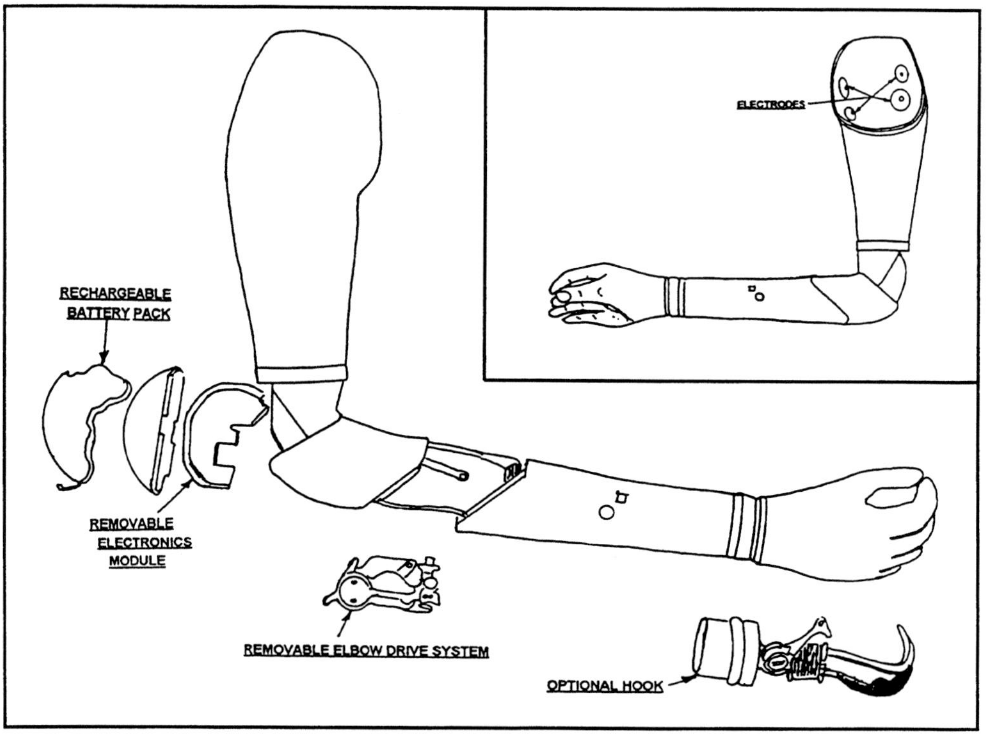


Figure 92. The Utah Elbow (8).The battery pack is located within the elbow unit and the elbow drive mechanism is located in the forearm unit. The easily removed components and interchangeable features make servicing easier and eliminate the need for the amputee to be without use of the prosthesis while major repairs are taking place. Courtesy of Motion Control, Inc.

Electrically-powered elbow units provide 135 degrees of flexion-extension in one plane. An adjustable friction turntable, similar to those used on the body-powered models, is used to permit manual positioning of the forearm in the vertical planes. In at least one design, the battery needed for a day's operation fits into the elbow itself and the motor for flexion-extension is located in the forearm (Figure 92).

Electrically-actuated locks that can be used in conjunction with body-powered elbow units are available when the amputee finds it difficult or impossible to provide the excursion needed to operate the alternating lock.

## Controls

Obviously, the key to successful use of externally-powered artificial arms is the control system. Controls may be proportional or they may be one or more simple on-off switches, or a combination of both. Control signals may be myoelectric (electrical signals generated by muscles as they contract) or biomechanical (such as relative motion between two body segments). Any combination of control sources may be employed to arrive at a system that provides the amputee with the arrangement that best fits his or her individual needs. Not surprisingly, a good deal of training is usually necessary when more than one control source is required. Proper sequencing of controls to obtain coordinated motion is difficult for many persons, and usually requires many hours of practice before efficient operation is achieved.

## Prescription

With the myriad combinations and permutations between electrically-powered units and body-powered units and systems, no consistent patterns of prescription seem to have evolved to date. Each clinical team, after a comprehensive evaluation of a patient, selects the components and control system that appears to be most useful for that patient. Fortunately, many of the components available from the different manufacturers are interchangeable, and thus permits prescriptions that are designed to best meet the individual needs of each patient (Figure 93). The end result may be, and often is, a hybrid between electric systems and body powered systems.

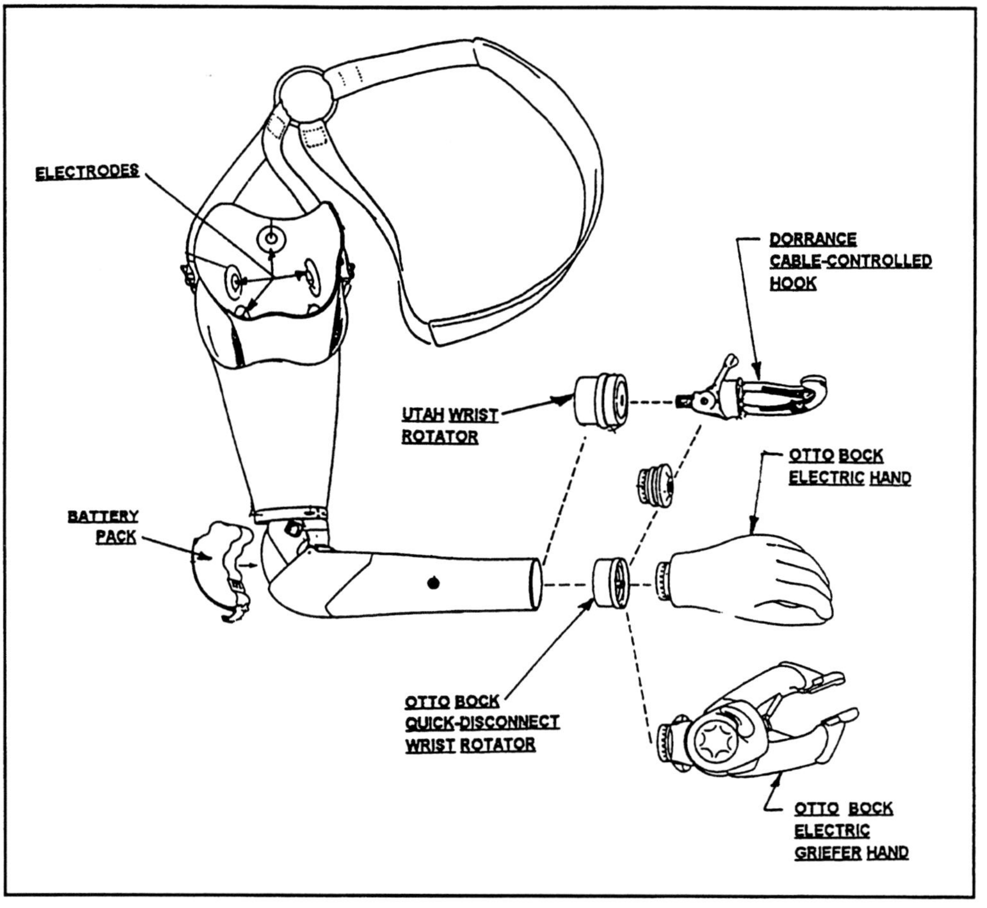


Figure 93. Graphic presentation of some of the possibilities for developing a prescription from modular, interchangeable components to provide a prosthesis that best meets the needs of individual amputees. Courtesy of Motion Control, Inc.

Because of the high costs of electrically-powered components, there are available methods for trials of some systems before the decision is made concerning the prescription of the definitive prosthesis.

# SPECIAL CONSIDERATIONS IN MANAGEMENT OF CHILD AMPUTEES

Children require artificial limbs as a result of either a congenital deficiency or anomaly, trauma, or disease. A true amputation caused by strangulation of a limb of an unborn child is rare, but not unheard of. A small percentage of limb deficiencies can be traced to genetic origins, but the vast majority seem to be the result of drug or other chemical ingestion by the mother, or an infectious disease such as rubella encountered by the mother during pregnancy. It is estimated that in about 40 percent of the cases with congenital deficiencies, more than one limb is involved.

To improve communication among those concerned with congenital deficiencies of limbs the Committee on Prosthetics Research and Development sponsored the development of a standard classification system, or nomenclature, in the 1960s and early 1970s (6). The International Society for Prosthetics and Orthotics, in the latter part of the 1970s, assumed the responsibility for making the system universally acceptable, and the result is a Standard issued relatively recently by the International Standards Organization (25).

The incidence of amputation due to trauma obviously increases as the child grows older, and the causes present no surprises–auto accidents, accidents in the home, accidents with lawnmowers and agriculture implements, gunshot wounds, etc. Surgeons should save as much length as medically and physiologically feasible.

Disarticulations are encouraged whenever possible rather than amputation at a higher level. Not only is the distal epiphysis preserved, thus allowing for continued growth of the long bones, but weightbearing is also allowed, suspension of the prosthesis is usually made easier, the stump is stronger, and more surface is provided over the stump so that unit pressures between stump and socket are reduced. However, it is not wise to disarticulate when a useful stump, usually transtibial, can be salvaged. The need for revisions at later dates to remove bone spurs that often form at the distal end is outweighed by the improved control provided by retaining as much skeletal structure and musculature and surface area as possible.

Because skin grafts are far more successful in children than in adult cases, it is possible to preserve more length in traumatic cases than might be the case with adults.

The function and appearance of children with anomalies such as vestigial extremities can sometimes be improved by surgical ablation or other procedures. Because the anomalies are so individual there is no well established set of procedures available and each case must be managed as the clinical team deems best for that individual case.

The disease that provides a reason for amputation of a limb in children in the majority of instances is cancer, but other problems such as infection can be a cause as well.

## PROSTHESES FOR CHILDREN

For the purpose of discussing the management of child amputees, the stages of development in children can be classified somewhat arbitrarily, as follows:

Birth - 12-18 months...........Infancy
18 months - 3 years.............Toddler Stage
3 years - 5-6 years...............Early Childhood
6 years - 12 years.................Middle Childhood
12 years - 16-17 years.........Adolescence

Beyond the age of 16 or 17, prescriptions for artificial limbs generally follow the guidelines that have been established for adults.

Congenital deficiencies, of course, account for all but a very few cases until adolescence. Management of children with absence of part of the lower limb or limbs at birth is usually straightforward. The child is fitted with an artificial leg as soon as he or she shows signs of wanting to walk. Children are very adaptable, and if the prosthesis is not too uncomfortable, they will use it as efficiently as the design and fitting will permit. Unfortunately, there is little consensus concerning the management of the younger groups with upper limb deficiencies whether in one or both arms.

Most dissertations on child amputees remind the reader that children are not scaled down adults and require devices designed to meet the special needs of children, not only in appropriate sizes, but also function. This, of course, is true, and there are available many components designed especially for children, especially for those with upper limb deficiencies.

## Bony Overgrowth

The major complication of amputation in children is bony overgrowth. The cause remains obscure, but it has been shown conclusively to be an additive phenomenon (36,37). Usually, a bursa is formed over the bony outgrowth, and if neglected, may proceed to skin penetration and a low-grade infection. This phenomenon is much more common in transhumeral and transtibial stumps as the epiphyses are more active in the proximal humerus and proximal tibia than say, in the proximal femur.

The most common method of treating bony overgrowth is resection of sufficient bone to allow adequate coverage with soft tissue.

Marquardt (36,37) developed a procedure styled as autogenous stump capping, to convert a metaphyseal or diaphyseal transverse deficiency amputation stump into a kind of disarticulation stump while successfully stopping bony overgrowth.

## Lower–Limb Prostheses

It is unlikely that anyone disagrees with the concept of fitting a child with a lower-limb prosthesis as soon as he or she shows signs of wanting to walk, sometimes as soon as eight or nine months. The child with an intact knee joint presents very little problem. When knee function is not present, it is usual practice to provide initially a prosthesis without joints. The gait will be ungainly, but it is normal for all children to walk with a wide-based gait until about five years old. Suspension of the prosthesis by a belt or harness is usually necessary. Articulated joints can be introduced at about three or four. Knee joints that can be locked manually are generally used to make the transition easier.

The rapid growth, both longitudinal and circumferential, usually found in children requires almost constant attention if proper fit and thus comfort and function are to be maintained. Circumferential growth can be compensated for over relatively short periods by making the socket slightly oversize and using several layers of prosthetic socks that can be removed one at a time as growth takes place. An alternative is use of a "triple wall" socket which consists of nesting sockets separated by a plastic film so that the inner two can be removed one at a time as the stump increases in size circumferentially. Some longitudinal growth can be accommodated by using a molded distal pad about one-half inch thick that can be replaced from time to time with progressively thinner pads.

The use of "flexible" sockets, inner sockets of a flexible molded transparent plastic, supported by a rigid frame, generally make accommodations for growth easier.

Longitudinal growth of the contralateral leg can be accommodated most easily when modular, or "pylon," prostheses are used, and the length can be increased easily by simply replacing the pylon with a slightly longer tube.

Alignment of the lower limb prosthesis for growing children is somewhat different for children than for the mature patient, and is best handled by a prosthetist with special training in this area.

Child amputees are notoriously hard on their prostheses, a factor that must be taken seriously. It is gratifying to find that a child is so well adjusted to being an amputee that he wears out his or her prosthesis quickly, but it is frustrating to all concerned when frequent repairs are required. For this reason, the prosthetist must try to provide a durable prosthesis that is not too heavy, sometimes a most difficult task.

Most children will not be concerned about appearance, or "cosmesis," until puberty, at which time every effort should be made to provide a prosthesis that appears to be as normal as practicable. With lifelike covers and soft fillers over modular prostheses, this is a need that is not as difficult to meet as it once was, but its importance is not to be overlooked. However, many teenagers are very active in sports, and it may be necessary to make some compromises between cosmesis and durability.

Constant follow-up of the child amputee is mandatory if maximum success, indeed any degree of success, is to be achieved.

## Upper-Limb Prostheses

For many reasons, there is little consensus on the management of children with congenital deficiencies of the upper limb. The primary reason, however, is that no comprehensive follow-up program for evaluation of results over a twenty-year period has been carried out. Such a program would be difficult and expensive and may be impractical, but more could be done than is now the case in improving the current knowledge of what works for whom.

For many years it was thought best to wait until the child was of school age before provision of an upper limb prosthesis. This approach, spurred by the availability of terminal devices designed especially for infants, was reversed and encouraging results seemed to be obtained when fittings occurred as soon as the child, especially those with only one side affected, was able to sit unaided. This is generally considered good practice for unilateral cases but should not be carried to extremes. Arguments can be made that it is best for fitting to be delayed until the child has reached the stage when he or she communicates well enough to participate actively in a training program. Many unilateral child amputees will use a prosthesis, sometimes adroitly, for several years, discard it at some point, only to express a desire for a hand as they become teenagers. They may or may not continue to use a prosthesis as an adult.

In some quarters, when both arms were affected, use of the feet to perform some functions normally assigned to hands was discouraged. The current practice seems to be to allow the child to develop naturally without and with prostheses, rather than forcing him or her to comply with some system thought by well-intentioned clinicians (and parents) to be the best for the child. Anecdotal reports of the experiences of the so-called Thalidomide children in Canada and the United Kingdom indicate that most of these children who were given extraordinary attention, especially in reference to prostheses, believe they would have made faster progress in becoming independent if they had been allowed to develop more naturally rather than being urged to use complicated gadgetry that was often uncomfortable and caused more trouble than it was worth.

The management of children with upper limb deficiencies has become even more complicated with the ready availability of externally-powered prostheses, especially those controlled by use of electromyographic signals. These systems have been promoted rather aggressively by some, but it is not at all clear what the overall results are.

## Conclusion

Still another complicating factor in management of the child amputee, whether due to congenital defects, trauma, or disease, but especially when congenital defects are the cause, is the parents. Most, naturally, are distraught and many feel guilty when there is no reason to be. Many parents feel that they are alone with the problem and justifiably have attitudes that require an experienced team to handle adequately.

Except for psychological attitudes, children with amputations caused by trauma or disease have most of the same problems as those who have been affected since birth. There is a wide range of devices, mostly scaled down designs originally intended for adult use, that are available for use by children as they mature through school age. Some will find use of a prosthesis satisfying; some will use prostheses for sports or special occasions; some will use prostheses during certain phases of maturation; others will prefer not to use a prosthesis at all. Each case must be handled on a highly individualistic basis.

For detailed discussions of all aspects of managing child amputees the reader is referred to "Part V: The Child Amputee" in *Atlas of Limb Prosthetics* (Bowker, J.H. and Michael, J., eds.) published in 1992 by Mosby-Year Book.

# SPECIAL CONSIDERATIONS IN MANAGEMENT OF ELDERLY AMPUTEES

Persons who have had amputations before the end of middle age seem to progress into the later stages of life with no more difficulty than the average person. However, when amputation occurs in later life, the cause is usually a circulatory problem that, more often than not, is accompanied by other physical problems, such as poor eyesight, poor balance, and weak musculature, that can severely affect rehabilitation. For many years, fitting such patients was considered unwise because such a small number of cases seemed to derive much benefit from a prosthesis. Furthermore, it was thought by many that ambulation would put more stress on the contralateral limb than need be, thus accelerating the need for a second amputation. However, it has been shown that use of crutches requires more energy than use of artificial limbs, especially when amputation is carried out below the knee, and most elderly patients can benefit from using an artificial leg. A rule of thumb is that if a lower limb amputee can master crutch walking or use a "walker" effectively, he or she should be provided with a prosthesis. This measure should be used with discretion because in some instances patients who did not meet either of these requirements have gone on to become successful users of artificial legs. Most clinic teams hold the view that if the prosthesis increases the patient's independence around the house or nursing home, the effort is fully warranted. With a very few exceptions, every lower limb amputee should be given the option of using a prosthesis.

In the Medicare Classification System (pg.78)(54), most elderly patients with transfemoral amputations fall into Level 1 (The ability or potential to use a prosthesis for transfers or ambulation on level surfaces at fixed cadence–typical of the limited and unlimited household ambulator). Most elderly amputees who have an intact knee will fall into Level 2 (The ability or potential for ambulation to traverse low level environmental barriers such as curbs, stairs, or uneven surfaces

–typical of the limited community ambulator). Thus prescriptions for prostheses that will be paid for by the Medicare program limits Level 1 patients to the use of a SACH Foot or a Single-Axis Foot and forbids the use of either hydraulic or pneumatic knee units, while Level 2 patients are allowed more sophisticated feet but not allowed hydraulic or pneumatic knee units. There exists considerable controversy about these limits that are yet to be resolved.

The elderly amputee should be fitted as soon as possible after surgery to avoid such complications as the development of muscle contractures. The availability of adjustable modular prostheses and the use of either plaster-of-paris or plastic sockets makes early fitting of a provisional prosthesis practical. Under carefully controlled conditions, many elderly amputees have benefited from immediate postoperative fitting, but general practice consists of providing a temporary or preparatory prosthesis as soon as the sutures are removed.

The weight of the prosthesis is even more important in the case of elderly amputees than it is for most younger amputees. Extreme care must be used in fitting so as to protect scars and skin grafts apt to be present from previous operations due to vascular surgery.

Suction sockets demand more strength and dexterity to don than elderly transfemoral amputees usually have, and therefore are seldom prescribed. Instead a slightly looser fitting, anatomically-shaped socket worn with a prosthetic sock and suspended with a Silesian Bandage is usually used.

For the elderly transtibial amputee, the PTB, or one of its variations, is applicable. When mediolateral stability of the knee presents a problem, it may be necessary to resort to a thigh lacer and side joints.

Very little, if any, changes in the prostheses normally used for ankle and knee disarticulations, respectively, are required.

# TRAINING AND "EDUCATION" OF THE AMPUTEE

Although some amputees, especially young persons with amputations at lower levels, might perform well without instruction in use of a prosthesis, these are exceptions, and for the amputee to derive the maximum benefit from the prosthesis, he or she usually requires a good deal of training. There have been instances in the past where amputees served as trainers for other amputees, but this is rare today. Lower-limb amputees are almost universally trained by physical therapists, while the upper-limb amputees are the domain of the occupational therapists (3,22). While the prosthetist must give the amputee the first set of instructions to walk or operate an artificial limb as the fitting process takes place, it is important that the therapist be involved as soon as possible, and obviously the more coordination there is between therapist and prosthetist, the better the process. It is all important that the therapist monitor closely the condition of the stump and other parts of the body to make sure that the fit, aligment, or function of the prosthesis is not causing problems that need to be corrected.

Other objectives of the training program are instruction in donning and doffing the prosthesis, recovery from a fall, caring for the stump and prosthesis, and use of crutches and canes when necessary.

Aside from teaching the amputee to use a prosthesis efficiently and intelligently, the therapist is responsible also for the physical conditioning of the user and instruction in exercises and behavior that will prevent the formation of contractures and encourage the development and maintenance of maximum range of motion of all joints of the body.

The prosthetist should emphasize to the patient that like all mechanical devices, good maintenance practices not only lenghten the life of a prosthesis but also help the prosthesis to provide maximum function. Also, the lower limb amputee needs to be warned of the dangers and difficulties involved in wearing the wrong type of shoe or shoes with worn heels, and encouraged to return to the prosthetist for maintenance on a schedule and should any problems arises visit the prosthetist as soon as possible.

For lower-limb amputees, there are available inexpensive booklets that many prosthetists provide to their patients that reinforce the oral instructions (42,43).

## RECOMMENDED READING

*Atlas of Limb Prosthetics-Surgical, Prosthetic, and Rehabilitation Principles* (2nd ed.) (John H. Bowker and John W. Michael, eds.), American Academy of Orthopaedic Surgeons, Mosby Year Book, St. Louis, 1992.

*Amputation: Surgical Practice and Patient Management* (G. Murdoch and A.Bennett Wilson, Jr. eds.), Butterworth-Heinemann, Oxford, England 1996.

# APPENDIX A
# ORGANIZATIONS CONCERNED PRIMARILY WITH REHABILITATION OF THE AMPUTEE

**American Orthotic and Prosthetic Association**
**American Board for Certification in Prosthetics and Orthotics**
**American Academy of Orthotists and Prosthetists**

During World War I, prosthetists and orthotists in the U.S. formed the Artificial Limb Manufacturers Association, which was operated largely on an informal basis until 1946, when a full-time executive director was employed, and the name was changed to the Orthopedic Appliances and Limb Manufacturers Association. The OALMA served not only as a trade association, but also as an academic institution in that it promoted educational activities and technical publications. Members of OALMA, with assistance from the American Academy of Orthopaedic Surgeons, created in 1948-9 the American Board for Certification of the Prosthetic and Orthopaedic Appliance Industry, now The American Board for Certification in Orthotics and Prosthetics, which certifies the credentials for both individuals and facilities. To carry the responsibility for the academic side of Prosthetics and Orthotics, the American Academy of Orthotists and Prosthetists was formed in 1970. Today the three groups work together closely in improving the practice of prosthetics and orthotics.

AOPA and AAOP publish jointly the quarterly *Journal of Prosthetics and Orthotics.*

**The International Society for Prosthetics and Orthotics**

For many years following World War II, the International Society for the Rehabilitation of the Disabled promoted progress in prosthetics and orthotics through a Committee on Prostheses, Braces, and Technical Aids. Largely through the efforts of Knud Jansen, an orthopaedic surgeon in Denmark, the activities of the Committee grew to the point that, with the blessing of the ISRD, the International Society for Prosthetics and Orthotics as a organization separate form the ISRD was founded in 1970. With headquarters in Copenhagen and a large membership, the ISPO has been a very positive influence on progress in research and clinical practice throughout the world. An International Conference is held every three years, and in addition to special reports on technical conferences, the Society publishes three times a year the technical journal, *Prosthetics and Orthotics International.*

**Association of Children's Orthotic-Prosthetic Clinics**

A small but significant part of the program of the Committee on Prosthetics Research and Development of the National Academy of Sciences was the Childrens Prosthetics Clinics Program. Begun in the 1950s to promote research and development in prostheses for children and the establishment of clinics devoted to child amputees, the program grew over the years to a point where a more formal organization of clinics and research groups was needed. Criteria for participation were developed and many clinics throughout the country applied and were accepted for membership. Meetings were held annually and communication was augmented by a small monthly publication, *The Interclinic Information Bulletin.* With the dissolution of the CPRD in 1976, the participating clinics, after a short hiatus, organized themselves into a self-sustaining group called the Association of Children's Prosthetic-Orthotic Clinics (ACPOC). ACPOC is currently comprised of more than 80 clinic teams throughout the United States and Canada, conducts a scientific meeting annually, and publishes *The Journal of the Association of Children's Orthotic-Prosthetic Clinics.*

**Amputee Coalition of America**

Through the years, there have been sporadic attempts to form support groups for amputees. Some flourished for relatively brief periods, only to eventually fade away for one or more reasons. By the late 1980s, though, a sufficient number of local groups were in existence to warrant the formation of a national leadership group. Spearheaded by a nurse, Mary Point Novotny, herself an amputee, the Amputee Coalition of America was created in 1990 to bring together the various local groups concerned with improving the quality of life for amputees through education of amputees, research personnel, clinical personnel, administrators, and the general public. The ACA has been eminently successful during the past decade. It has established a center for information about amputations and amputees and publishes a very informative magazine, In-Motion, six times a year.

## STANDARDS

Until the early 1970s, very little concern was given to the establishment of any kind of standards in the field of external limb prostheses. Upon the recommendation of ISPO, the International Standards Organization created a technical committee, ISO/TC 168, to develop standards in three areas of limb prosthetics: Nomenclature, Description of Amputation Stumps, and Physical Standards. Work of this sort is inherently slow, but progress has been made over the years. A standard vocabulary and nomenclature for amputation levels and congenital limb deficiencies has been established (25). Standard methods for describing amputation stumps and prostheses have been adopted (26,27,28,29). Standards for structural integrity and quality of manufacture are in draft form.

# APPENDIX B

# EDUCATION AND TRAINING PROGRAMS IN THE U.S.A.

## ORTHOTIC AND PROSTHETIC PRACTITIONER PROGRAMS

### Key

1. Baccalaureate Degree Program
2. Postbaccalaureate Certificate Program
3. Accredited by Commision on Accreditation of Allied Health Programs

***California***

California State University
Dominquez Hills
1000 E. Victoria Street
Carson, CA 90747
1,2,3

***Connecticut***

Newington Certificate Program
181 E. Cedar Street
Newington, CT 06111
2,3

***Illinois***

Northwestern University Prosthetic-Orthotic Center
345 E. Superior Street
Chicago, IL 60611
3

***Minnesota***

Century College
O&P Programs
3300 Century Avenue, N.
White Bear Lake, MN 55110
2

***New Jersey***

Rurgers University
Orthotic and Prosthetic Laboratory
Department of Biomechanical Engineering
Piscataway, NJ 08855-0909
3

***Texas***

Southwestern Medical Center
University of Texas
School of Allied Health Sciences
Orthotics and Prosthetics Programs
6011 Harry Hines Blvd.
Dallas, TX 75235-9091
1

***Washington***

University of Washington
School of Medicine
Division of Orthotics and Prosthetics
Seattle, WA 98195
1

## ORTHOTIC AND PROSTHETIC TECHNICIAN PROGRAMS

**Key**

1. Associate Degree Program
2. Certificate Program

***Minnesota***

Century College
Orthotics and Prosthetics Programs
3300 Century Avenue, N.
White Bear Lake, MN 55110
1,2

***Pennsylvania***

Median School of Allied Health Careers
125 Seventh Street
Pittsburgh, PA 15222
1,2

***Washington***

Spokane Falls Community College
W. 3410 Fort George Wright Drive
MS 3020
Spokane, WA 99204-5288
1,2

# REFERENCES


1. American Academy of Orthopaedic Surgeons. Historical developments of artificial limbs. In *Orthopaedic Appliances Atlas*, Vol. 2, J.W. Edwards, Ann Arbor, 1960.
2. American Orthotic and Prosthetic Association, *The illustrated guide to orthotics and prosthetics*, 1992.
3. Atkins, Diane, Adult upper limb prosthetic training. Chapter 11 in *Atlas of Limb Prosthetics*, (2nd ed.) Mosby, 1992.
4. Barth, D.G., Shumaker, L., & Sienko-Thomas, S. Gait analysis and energy costs of below-knee amputees wearing six different prosthetic feet. *J.Pros.Orth.*, 1992:4 (2)63-75.
5. Blomhke, F. Otto Bock Prosthetic Compendium - Lower Extremity Prostheses. Schiele & Schon. Berlin 1989.
6. Bunnell, S. The management of the nonfunctional hand - Reconstruction vs pros thesis. *Artif. Limbs, 4:1,* 76-102, Spring, 1957.
7. Blomhke, F. Otto Bock Prosthetic Compendium - Upper Extremity Prostheses. Schiele & Schon. Berlin, 1992.
8. Burgess, E.M., Hittenberger, D.A., Forsgren, S.M., & Sindh, D. The Seattle foot–A design for active sports: Preliminary studies. *Orth.&Pros., 37:1,*. 25-31, 1983.
9. Campbell, J.W., & Childs, C.W. The SAFE foot. *Orth.&Pros.*, 34:3 3-16, Sept. 1980.
10. CaTech, Inc., Centerville, OH.
11. Cascade Orthopedic Supply, Inc., Chester, CA.
12. Condie, D. N., & Stills, M.L. Prosthetic and orthotic management (Partial Foot Amputations). In *Atlas of Limb Prosthetics* (2nd ed.). American Academy of Orthopaedic Surgeons. Mosby, 1992.
13. de Fries, J. Conventional 4-bar linkage knee mechanisms: A strength-weakness analysis. *J. Rehab. R&D*, 32:1, pp. 36-42, Feb. 1995.
14. Donovan, R.D., Pritham, C., & Wilson, A.B. (Eds). Report of workshops–International wworkshop on above-knee fitting and alignment, May 1987, and Workshop on teaching materials for above-knee socket variants, October, 1987, *Int. Soc. Pros.&Orth.,* 1987.
15. Dorrance, D.W. U.S. Patent No. 1,042.413, issued October 29, 1912.
16. Eberhart, Howard D., Inman, Verne T., & Bresler, Boris. The principal elements in human locomotion. In Klopsteg & Wilson's Human Limbs and Their Substitutes. McGraw-Hill, 1954, reissued by Hafner Press, 1968.
17. Ferrier Coupler Inc., North Branch, MI.
18. Fillauer, C.E., Pritham, C.H., & Fillauer, K.D.. Evolution and development of the silicone suction socket (3S) for below-knee prostheses. *J. Pros. & Orth., 1*:2, 92-103, 1989.

19. Fletcher, M.J. The upper-extremity armentarium. *Artif. Limbs,* pp 15-24, May 1954.
20. Flex-Foot, Laguna Hills, CA.
21. Fryer, C.M. Harnessing and controls for body-poweredd devices. In *Atlas of Limb Prosthetics* (2nd ed.). American Academy of Orthopaedic Surgeons, Mosby, 1992.
22. Gailey, Robert S., & Clark, Curtis R. Physical therapy management of adult lower limb amputees In *Atlas of Limb Prosthetics* (2nd ed.). American Academy of Orthopaeclic Surgeons, Mosby, 1992.
23. Hosmer Dorrance Corp., Catalog, 1992. Campbell, CA.
24. Inman, Verne T. Conservation of energy in ambulation. *Bull. Pros. Research, BPR 10-9,* 26-35, Spring 1968.
25. International Standards Organization, *ISO 8548-1, Prosthetics and Orthotics–Limb deficiencies–Method of describing limb deficiencies at birth.* Geneva, 1989.
26. International Standards Organization, *ISO 8548-2, Prosthetics and Orthotics - Limb deficiencies - Method of describing lower limb amputation stumps.* Geneva, 1993.
27. International Standards Organization, *ISO 8548-3, Prosthetics and Orthotics–Limb deficiencies–Method of describing upper limb stumps.* Geneva, 1993.
28. International Standards Organization, *ISO 8549, Prosthetics and Orthotics - General terms for external limb prostheses and external orthoses.* Geneva 1989.
29. International Standards Organization, *ISO 8549-2, Terms relating to external limb prostheses and wearers of these prostheses.* Geneva, 1989.
30. Kay, H., & Newman, J.D., Relative incidences of new amputations. *Ortho. & Pros.* 29:2, 3-16, June, 1975.
31. Kingsley Manufacturing Co., Costa Mesa, CA.
32. Kristinsson, O. Flexible above-knee socket made from low density polyethylene suspended by a weight transmitting frame. *Ortho. & Pros., 37:*2, 25-37, 1983.
33. Liberty Technology, Hopkinton, MA.
34. Lyquist, E. The OHC kneee disarticulation prosthesis. *Ortho. & Pros., 30:2,* 27-28, June 1976.
35. Marks, A.A. *Manual of Artificial Limbs.* A.A. Marks, New York, 1906.
36. Marquardt, E. The Heidelberg experience. In *Comprehensive Management of the Upper Limb Amputee* (D.Y. Adkins & R.H. Meier, III, Eds.). Springer, pp210-252, 1991
37. Marquardt, E. The multiple limb deficient child. In *Atlas of Limb Prosthetics* (2nd ed.). American Academy of Orthopaedic Surgeons, Mosby, pp 839-884, 1992
38. Mauch Laboratories, Inc., Dayton, OH.
39. Motion Control, Inc., Salt Lake City, UT.
40. M+IND, Seattle, WA. (Now Seattle Limb Systems).
41. Murdoch, G., & Wilson, A.B. A Short History (Of Prosthetics), in *A Primer on Amputations and Artificial Limbs.* Charles C Thomas, 1998.
42. Muilenburg, Alvin, & Wilson, A.Bennett. *A Manual for Above-Knee (Trans-Femoral) Amputees* (5th ed.). Rehabilitation Press, Topping, VA, 1996.
43. Muilenburg, Alvin, & Wilson, A.Bennett. *A Manual for Below-Knee (Trans-Tibial) amputees* (5th ed.). Rehabilitation Press, Topping, VA, 1996

44. Nielsen, D.H., Shurr, D.G., Golden, J.C., & Meier, K. Comparison of energy cost and gait efficiency during ambulation in below-knee amputees using different prosthetic feet: A preliminary report. *J.Pros & Orth., 1*:1, 24-31, 1988.
45. Ohio Willow Wood Co., Mt. Sterling, OH.
46. Otto Bock Orthopedic Industries, INc., Catalog. Minneapolis, MN.
47. Pentland, J.A., & Wasilieff, A. An above-elbow suction socket. *Ortho. & Pros., 27*:2, 36-40, June 1973.
48. Pursley, R.J. Harness Patterns for upper-extremity prostheses. *Artif. Limbs, 2*:3, 26-60, September 1955.
49. Radcliffe, C.W. Four-bar linkage prosthetic knee mechanisms: Kinematics, alignment, and prescription criteria. *Pros. & Orth. Int., 18*:159-193, 1994.
50. Radocy, B. Upper-limb prosthetic adaptations for sports and recreation. In *Atlas of Limb Prosthetics* (2nd ed.). American Academy of Orthopaedic Surgeons, Mosby, 1992.
51. Ralston, H.J. Energy-speed relation and optimal speed during level walking. *Int. Zangew Physiol., 17*:277-283, 1958.
52. Saunders, J.B.deC.M., Inman, V.T., & Eberhart, H.D. The major determinants in normal and pathological gait. *J.Bone & Joint Surg.*, 35-A:543-558, July 1953.
53. Schlesinger, G. Die milarbeit des ingenieurs bei de durchbildung der ersatzglieder, Verein. Deutsch Ingen., *Berlin Ztschr, 61*:6, 1917.
54. Social Security Administration (U.S.). *DMERC Medicare Advisory*. U.S. Government, pp94-214 through 92-219, December 1994.
55. Taylor, C.L. The biomechanics of the normal and of the amputated upper extremity. In *Klopsteg & Wilson's Human Limbs and Their Substitutes.* McGraw-Hill, New York, 1954, reprinted by Hafner Press, 1968.
56. Torburn, L., Powers, C., Guiterrez., & Perry, J. Energy expenditure during ambulation in dysvascular and traumatic below-knee amputees. A comparison of five prosthetic feet. *J. Rehab. R&D, 32*:3, 111-119, May 1995.
57. T.R.S., Inc., Boulder, CO.
58. U.S. Manufacturing Co., Pasadena, CA. Catalog, 1995.
59. Variety Ability Systems, Inc., Scarborough, Canada.
60. Wilson, A.B., History of amputation surgery and prosthetics, In *Atlas of Limb Prosthetics*, (2nd ed.). American Academy of Orthopedic Surgeons, Mosby 1992.
61. Wilson, A.B. The prosthetics and orthotics program. *Artif. Limbs, 14*:2, 1970.

# SUBJECT INDEX

**R**

# ILLUSTRATIONS INDEX